Milady's Standard
State Exam Review for Cosmetology

Edited by Sharon MacGregor

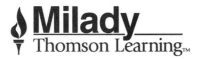

Milady
Thomson Learning™

Foreword

Milady's Standard State Exam Review for Cosmetology has been revised to follow very closely the type of cosmetology questions most frequently used by states and by the national testing, conducted under the auspices of the National-Interstate Council of State Boards of Cosmetology.

This review book is designed to be of major assistance to students in preparing for the state license examinations. In addition, its regular use in the classroom will serve as an important aid in the understanding of all subjects taught in cosmetology schools and required in the practice of cosmetology.

The exclusive concentration on multiple-choice test items reflects the fact that all state board examinations and national testing examinations are confined to this type of question.

Questions on the state board examinations in different states will not be exactly like these and may not touch upon all the information covered in this review. But students who diligently study and practice their work as taught in the classroom and who use this book for test preparation and review should receive higher grades on both classroom and license examinations.

Contents

Your Professional Image

1. Personal grooming is an extension of:
   a) public hygiene
   b) personal hygiene
   c) personal development
   d) professional ethics

   B

2. The science that deals with the daily maintenance of health by the individual is:
   a) good grooming
   b) self-preservation
   c) personal hygiene
   d) personal development

   C

3. Good posture prevents fatigue and creates an image of:
   a) superiority
   b) personal hygiene
   c) confidence
   d) good grooming

   C

4. The body may be kept clean by the regular use of:
   a) deodorants
   b) soap and water
   c) moisturizers
   d) germicides

   B

5. Body odors can be prevented by regular bathing and use of:
   a) a protective outer garment
   b) astringents
   c) germicides
   d) deodorants

   D

6. Maintaining healthy teeth and keeping the breath sweet is known as:
   a) gargling
   b) oral hygiene
   c) mouth deodorization
   d) mouth lubrication

   B

7. To keep your teeth in a good, healthy condition, it is necessary to maintain regular:
   a) physicals
   b) oral exercise
   c) use of deodorants
   d) dental care

   D

8. Bad or offensive breath may be treated and minimized by:
   a) gargling with an astringent
   b) throat lozenges
   c) drinking water
   d) rinsing with mouthwash

   D

9. Rest and relaxation are necessary to prevent:
   a) fatigue
   b) poor eating habits
   c) poor oral hygiene
   d) body odors

   A

10. Overexertion and lack of rest tend to drain the body of its:
    a) supply of sebum
    b) efficiency
    c) perspiration
    d) blood supply

    B

11. One of the major elements required for good health is:
    a) a well-balanced diet
    b) adequate makeup
    c) proper clothing
    d) personal disinfection

    A

12. Factors that may be considered health hazards are:
    a) a single restroom
    b) impure air and food
    c) leaky faucets
    d) streaked salon mirrors

    A

13. One of the best advertisements of an efficiently run salon is a cosmetologist who is:
    a) well groomed
    b) well paid
    c) youthful in appearance
    d) physically fit

    A

14. An important consideration in personal hygiene is:
    a) good posture
    b) efficiency
    c) ethical conduct
    d) cleanliness

    D

15. The use of good speech is vital to the art of:
    a) literature
    b) fashion
    c) conversation
    d) grooming

    C

16. The cosmetologist who practices correct posture will find that it helps reduce:
    a) skin discoloration
    b) body fatigue
    c) weight gain
    d) muscular coordination

    B

17. For a good standing posture, keep the head up, chin level with the floor, chest up, shoulders relaxed, and:
    a) lower abdomen out   c) lower abdomen flat
    b) knees close together   d) feet wide apart

    C

18. For a good sitting posture, keep the feet and:
    a) arms close together   c) chin out
    b) knees close together   d) chest relaxed

    B

19. For a comfortable sitting posture, keep the soles of the feet:
    a) on the floor   c) extended
    b) crossed   d) elevated

    A

20. The muscles of the body are kept in good condition by:
    a) tonics   c) conditioners
    b) moisturizers   d) exercise

    D

21. In order to give the body support and balance and to help maintain good posture, the cosmetologist should wear:
    a) slip-on shoes   c) low-heeled shoes
    b) cushioned loafers   d) fashionable shoes

    C

22. Personal hygiene includes all of the following EXCEPT:
    a) oral hygiene   c) cleaning your nails
    b) bathing or showering   d) wearing the latest fashions

    D

23. To avoid back strain while working, sit:
    a) toward the back of   c) on the forward part of the
       the chair   chair
    b) to one side of the chair d) with legs crossed

    A

24. A well-groomed cosmetologist does not wear:
    a) makeup   c) cologne
    b) obtrusive jewelry   d) a watch

    B

25. Public hygiene is also known as:
    a) personal hygiene   c) sanitation
    b) sterilization   d) disinfection

    C

26. Skills that include listening, manner of speaking, and your voice are all a part of:
    a) physical presentation
    b) professionalism
    c) communication
    d) management skills

    B

27. Rules involving professional ethics for cosmetology include all of the following EXCEPT:
    a) respecting others' beliefs and rights ✓
    b) being loyal to your employer, manager, and coworkers ✓
    c) treating everyone honestly and fairly ✓
    d) getting adequate rest and nutrition

    D

28. Thoughtfulness of others is considered to be the foundation of:
    a) good grooming
    b) personality development
    c) vitality
    d) courtesy

    B

29. To be successful, it is most important to avoid body odor and:
    a) the use of bar soap
    b) punctuality
    c) bad breath
    d) good grooming

    C

30. Good topics for salon conversation should be:
    a) political
    b) debatable
    c) religious
    d) noncontroversial

    D

31. A smile of greeting and a word of welcome are two personality characteristics that reflect:
    a) liveliness
    b) graciousness
    c) a good education
    d) a sense of humor

    B

32. Courtesy is the key to:
    a) effective negotiating
    b) success
    c) booking appointments
    d) outsmarting others

    B

33. One of the cosmetologist's most important personal assets is his/her:
    a) personality
    b) physical appearance
    c) wardrobe
    d) financial standing

    A

34. Good conversation involves the use of a pleasant voice, good choice of words, intelligence, charm, and:
    a) grooming
    b) education
    c) personality
    d) repetition

    C

35. Proper conduct in relation to employer, clients, and coworkers is called professional:
    a) personality
    b) ethics
    c) courtesy
    d) honesty

    B

36. Repeating gossip will cause loss of the patron's:
    a) attention
    b) gratuity
    c) confidence
    d) interest

    D

37. An important attribute of good professional ethics is:
    a) personal appearance
    b) loyalty
    c) personal hygiene
    d) intelligence

    B

38. All clients must be treated honestly and fairly, without any demonstration of:
    a) flattery
    b) courtesy
    c) humor
    d) favoritism

    D

39. Clients will respect and be loyal to a cosmetologist who is:
    a) fashionable
    b) funny
    c) talkative
    d) courteous

    D

40. The true professional treats the feelings and rights of others:
    a) without tact
    b) with familiarity
    c) with respect
    d) with disdain

    C

41. The wise and successful cosmetologist is most often a good:
    a) storyteller
    b) conversationalist
    c) listener
    d) friend

    C

42. It is important to handle clients with:
    a) good humor
    b) tact
    c) simple language
    d) facts only

    B

5

43. Clients' complaints and grievances should be treated promptly and:
    a) discreetly
    b) with a cash refund
    c) with a manager present
    d) in person

    A

Bacteriology

1. The scientific study of microorganisms is known as:
   - a) pathology
   - b) biology
   - c) bacteriology
   - d) genealogy

   C

2. Bacteria are one-celled microorganisms of:
   - a) animal origin
   - b) vegetable origin
   - c) mineral origin
   - d) chemical origin

   B

3. A type of pathogenic bacteria is the:
   - a) parasite
   - b) saprophyte
   - c) pathotyte
   - d) cilia

   A

4. Pathogenic bacteria produce:
   - a) health
   - b) beneficial effects
   - c) antitoxins
   - d) disease

   D

5. Harmful bacteria are referred to as:
   - a) saprophytes
   - b) pathogenic
   - c) nonpathogenic
   - d) protozoa

   B

6. Nonpathogenic bacteria are:
   - a) harmful
   - b) cocci
   - c) harmless
   - d) disease producing

   C

7. Pathogenic bacteria are commonly known as:
   - a) spores
   - b) dust
   - c) germs
   - d) beneficial bacteria

   C

8. Syphilis is caused by a _____ organism.
   a) bacilli
   b) spirilla
   c) diplococci
   d) cocci

   _____

9. Cocci are bacteria with a:
   a) round shape
   b) rod shape
   c) corkscrew shape
   d) curved shape

   _____

10. Bacilli are bacteria with a:
    a) corkscrew shape
    b) round shape
    c) rod shape
    d) curved shape

    _____

11. Spirilla are bacteria with a:
    a) round shape
    b) corkscrew shape
    c) rod shape
    d) flat shape

    _____

12. Bacteria cells reproduce by simply dividing in:
    a) half
    b) quarters
    c) thirds
    d) eighths

    _____

13. Pustules and boils are infections containing:
    a) nonpathogenic organisms
    b) pathogenic organisms
    c) sebum
    d) ringworm

    _____

14. Bacteria are also known as:
    a) viruses
    b) fungi
    c) microbes
    d) verruca

    _____

15. Some forms of bacteria have the ability to move about with the aid of:
    a) flagella
    b) air movement
    c) moisture
    d) spores

    _____

16. The inactive phase in the life cycle of bacteria is known as the:
    a) pathogenic stage
    b) spore-forming stage
    c) mitosis stage
    d) nonpathogenic stage

    _____

17. A communicable disease is:
    a) not transferred from one person to another
    c) transmitted from one person to another
    b) prevented by vaccination
    d) caused by nonpathogenic bacteria _____

18. The common cold and other viruses are caused by:
    a) plant parasites
    c) animal parasites
    b) filterable viruses
    d) fungi _____

19. Bacteria are not harmed by disinfectants while in the:
    a) vegetative stage
    c) active stage
    b) spore-forming stage
    d) mitosis stage _____

20. Bacteria may enter the body through:
    a) dry skin
    c) broken skin
    b) moist skin
    d) oily skin _____

21. Resistance to disease is known as:
    a) superiority
    c) DNA
    b) immunity
    d) immunization _____

22. An example of a general infection is:
    a) a boil
    c) an epidemic
    b) syphilis
    d) a skin lesion _____

23. Organisms that live on other organisms without giving anything in return are known as:
    a) greedy
    c) diphtheria
    b) para-organisms
    d) parasites _____

24. Cosmetologists should not work on patrons if they have a:
    a) common cold
    c) keratoma
    b) carbuncle
    d) macule _____

25. Acquired immune deficiency syndrome attacks and destroys:
    a) the body's nerves
    c) only homosexuals
    b) the body's immune system
    d) needle users _____

26. AIDS is caused by:
    a) the HIV virus   c) lack of proper nutrition
    b) herpes   d) the flu   _____

27. The HIV virus may not be transferred by:
    a) bodily fluids   c) semen
    b) blood   d) coughing   _____

Decontamination and Infection Control

1. Surfaces of tools or other objects that are not free from dirt, oils, and microbes are:
   a) sterile
   b) contaminated
   c) pathogenic
   d) infected

   B

2. When disposing of contaminated wipes or cotton balls from a blood spill, they should be placed:
   a) in a trash receptacle
   b) in a towel
   c) outside in a garbage dumpster
   d) in a sealed plastic bag before disposing

   D

3. The three main levels of decontamination are sterilization, disinfection, and:
   a) clean
   b) contamination
   c) sanitation
   d) infection

   C

4. Removing pathogens and other substances from tools or surfaces is called:
   a) cleaning
   b) controlling
   c) scrubbing
   d) decontamination

   D

5. The level of decontamination not required in the salon is:
   a) sanitation
   b) sterilization
   c) decontamination
   d) cleaning

   B

6. Sterilization is used by:
   a) nail technicians
   b) surgeons
   c) cosmetologists
   d) maids

   B

7. Surfaces that may be sterilized are:
   a) nail plates
   b) non-porous surfaces
   c) wood
   d) skin

   B

8. Disinfection is one step below sterilization because it does *not*:
   a) remove oil
   b) kill microbes
   c) kill most organisms
   d) kill bacterial spores

   D

9. Instruments used to penetrate the skin may be:
   a) given to the client after use
   b) disposable instruments
   c) first washed in soap and water
   d) handled with tongs

   B

10. Disinfectants should never be used on human skin, hair, or nails because:
    a) they can stain skin
    b) damage can result
    c) they can lighten skin
    d) they are not strong enough

    B

11. An important number on a disinfectant label is the:
    a) bar code
    b) toll free number
    c) EPA registration number
    d) MSDS registration number

    C

12. OSHA was created to regulate and enforce:
    a) salon hazardous actions
    b) sanitary habitats
    c) sloppy household accidents
    d) safety and health standards

    D

13. Every product used in the cosmetology school or salon should have a/an:
    a) warranty
    b) opaque container
    c) MSDS
    d) EPA registration number

    C

14. Important information found on an MSDS includes:
    a) other uses of product
    b) storage requirements
    c) other suppliers of product
    d) resale value of product

     B

15. If a salon implement comes into contact with blood or body fluids, it should be cleaned and completely immersed in:
    a) alcohol
    b) an EPA-registered disinfectant that kills HIV-1 and Hepatitis B
    c) formalin
    d) an OSHA-registered antiseptic that retards airborne diseases

    B

16. A disinfectant that is "Formulated for Hospitals and Health Care Facilities" must be pseudomonacidal, bactericidal, fungicidal, and:
    a) pneumonicidal
    b) inexpensive
    c) virucidal
    d) easy to dilute for other uses _C_

17. Before soaking in a disinfectant, implements must be thoroughly:
    a) dry
    b) cleaned
    c) heated
    d) soaked _B_

18. The purpose of a wet sanitizer is to actually:
    a) disinfect
    b) sanitize
    c) sterilize
    d) store dirty implements _A_

19. The solution used in a wet sanitizer should be changed:
    a) whenever it looks cloudy
    b) weekly
    c) daily
    d) every other day _C_

20. When a client is accidentally cut with a sharp instrument, it is known as a/an:
    a) critical injury
    b) blood emergency
    c) accident
    d) blood spill _D_

21. Most quaternary ammonium compounds disinfect implements in:
    a) 5–10 seconds
    b) 5–10 minutes
    c) 2–5 minutes
    d) 10–15 minutes _D_

22. Phenolic disinfectants are used mostly for:
    a) rubber and plastic
    b) metal implements
    c) skin sanitization
    d) blood spills _B_

23. States requiring hospital disinfection do not allow the use of _____ for disinfection of implements:
    a) alcohol
    b) quats
    c) phenols
    d) antiseptics _A_

24. Two disinfectants used in the salon in the past, but since replaced by more advanced and effective technologies, are:
    a) quats & phenols
    b) phenols & bleach
    c) alcohol & quats
    d) alcohol & bleach _D_

13

25. The technical name for bleach is:
    a) sodium hydroxide
    b) sodium hypochlorite
    c) sodium chloride
    d) sodium hydroclorox

    B

26. Ultrasonic bath cleaners are an effective way to clean tiny crevices in implements only when used with:
    a) an effective disinfectant
    b) an effective astringent
    c) an ultrasonic surfactant
    d) stearyl alcohol

    A

27. Rather than using bar soaps, which can grow bacteria, you should provide:
    a) baby cleanser
    b) pump-type antibacterial soap
    c) alcohol wipes
    d) a wash cloth

    B

28. Properly disinfected implements should be stored in a/an:
    a) station drawer
    b) wet sanitizer
    c) open container on station
    d) disinfected and covered container

    D

29. The lowest level of decontamination is called sanitation or:
    a) rubbish removal
    b) sanitization
    c) sterilization
    d) infection control

    B

30. An example of sanitation is:
    a) boiling implements
    b) an autoclave
    c) washing your hands
    d) a bead sterilizer

    C

31. Two rules of universal precautions involve your personal hygiene and:
    a) your general health
    b) your attitude
    c) your personal appearance
    d) salon cleanliness

    D

32. Disinfectants should be stored in containers that are:
    a) labeled
    b) stabilized
    c) clear
    d) OSHA approved

    A

33. Before a surface is disinfected, it should be properly:
    a) painted
    b) cleaned
    c) scored
    d) dried

    B

34. Gloves should be worn when working with:
    a) antiseptics
    b) hot water
    c) disinfectants
    d) a bead sanitizer

    _C_

35. Sterilization may be accomplished by using a steam autoclave or:
    a) cool vapors
    b) rinsing with alcohol
    c) dry heat
    d) soaking in sterilizer acid

    _C_

Properties of the Hair and Scalp

1. The study of the hair is called:
   a) hairology
   b) dermatology
   c) trichology
   d) biology _____

2. The chief purposes of the hair are adornment and:
   a) sweat diversion
   b) oil reduction
   c) flattering appearance
   d) protection _____

3. Hair is not found on the palms of the hands, soles of the feet, lips, and:
   a) neck
   b) eyelids
   c) ankles
   d) wrists _____

4. Three types of hair on the body are classified as long hair, short or bristly hair, and:
   a) pigmented hair
   b) vellus
   c) cilia
   d) terminal hair _____

5. The technical term for eyelash hair is:
   a) cilia
   b) barba
   c) capilli
   d) supercilia _____

6. Hair is composed chiefly of:
   a) oxygen
   b) keratin
   c) melanin
   d) sulfur _____

7. The chemical composition of hair varies with its:
   a) thickness
   b) length
   c) color
   d) growth pattern _____

8. The two main divisions of the hair are the hair root and:
   a) hair shaft
   b) follicle
   c) papilla
   d) bulb
   _____

9. The hair root is located:
   a) above the skin surface
   b) below the skin surface
   c) under the cuticle
   d) within the cortex
   _____

10. The three main structures associated with the hair root are the follicle, the bulb, and:
    a) the hair stream
    b) the papilla
    c) the hair shaft
    d) the medulla
    _____

11. The hair root is encased by a tubelike depression in the skin known as the:
    a) bulb
    b) arrector pili
    c) papilla
    d) follicle
    _____

12. Follicles are set at an angle so the hair above the surface:
    a) flows to one side
    b) forms a cowlick
    c) does not fall out
    d) has volume
    _____

13. The club-shaped structure that forms the lower part of the hair root is the:
    a) arrector pili
    b) bulb
    c) papilla
    d) hair shaft
    _____

14. The papilla is located:
    a) below the medulla
    b) above the hair root
    c) at the bottom of the follicle
    d) at the skin surface
    _____

15. The small involuntary muscle attached to the underside of the follicle is known as the:
    a) erector muscle
    b) arrector pili
    c) gooseflesh flexor
    d) follicle tendon
    _____

16. Oil glands are also known as:
    a) suderiferous glands
    b) sebaceous glands
    c) endocrine glands
    d) follicle glands
    _____

17. The oily substance secreted from the oil glands is called:
    a) lymph
    b) melanosome
    c) humectous
    d) sebum
    _____

18. Oil glands are connected to:
    a) hair follicles
    b) arteries
    c) hair roots
    d) nerves
    _____

19. The three layers of the hair are the cuticle, cortex, and
    a) bulb
    b) medulla
    c) root
    d) shaft
    _____

20. The cuticle's scalelike cells protect:
    a) the scalp
    b) the root
    c) the inner structure of
       the hair
    d) the outside horny layer
    _____

21. Hair pigment is found in the _____ layer.
    a) cuticle
    b) medulla
    c) cortex
    d) pith
    _____

22. The innermost layer of the hair is referred to as the pith, marrow,
    or:
    a) cuticle
    b) medulla
    c) cortex
    d) protective layer
    _____

23. If hair is pulled out from the roots, it will:
    a) never grow again
    b) grow in gray
    c) grow in thicker
    d) grow again
    _____

24. If the papilla is destroyed, the hair will:
    a) never grow again
    b) grow in gray
    c) grow in thicker
    d) grow again
    _____

25. Eyebrows and eyelashes are replaced:
    a) daily
    b) monthly
    c) weekly
    d) every 4–5 months
    _____

26. The natural color of hair, its strength, and its texture depend mainly on:
    a) exposure to sunlight
    b) the follicle
    c) the cortex
    d) heredity
    _____

27. A person born with an absence of coloring matter in the hair shaft and no marked pigment coloring in the skin or irises of the eyes is a/an:
    a) vitiligo
    c) Caucasian
    b) melanin deficient
    d) albino
    _____

28. Gray hair:
    a) appears at age 40
    c) sheds easily
    b) multiplies with removal
    d) grows that way from the bulb
    _____

29. In most cases, gray hair is caused by:
    a) the natural aging process
    c) unnatural shock to the body
    b) type A personality
    d) albinism
    _____

30. Long, thick pigmented hair is known as:
    a) vellus
    c) terminal
    b) supercilia
    d) cilia
    _____

31. Vellus hair is:
    a) pigmented
    c) nonpigmented
    b) coarse
    d) curly
    _____

32. The three phases of hair growth are anagen, catagen, and:
    a) biogen
    c) active
    b) transitional
    d) telogen
    _____

33. The growing phase of hair growth is known as:
    a) anagen
    c) catagen
    b) biogen
    d) telogen
    _____

34. Hair grows approximately:
    a) 1" per month
    c) 1/4" per month
    b) 1/2" per month
    d) 1 1/4" per month
    _____

35. At any one time _____% of our hair is growing.
    a) 10
    c) 75
    b) 50
    d) 90
    _____

36. Hair continues to grow for a period of:
    a) 2–6 months
    c) 2–6 weeks
    b) 2–6 years
    d) 26 months
    _____

37. The transitional phase of hair growth is known as:
    a) anagen
    b) telogen
    c) biogen
    d) catagen

    _____

38. The transitional phase of hair growth lasts approximately:
    a) 1–2 days
    b) 1–2 months
    c) 1–2 weeks
    d) 1–2 years

    _____

39. During catagen the follicle:
    a) increases in volume
    b) thickens
    c) lengthens
    d) decreases in volume

    _____

40. The lower part of the _____ is destroyed during the transitional phase of the hair life cycle.
    a) hair root
    b) hair follicle
    c) hair bulb
    d) papilla

    _____

41. The resting phase of the hair growth cycle is known as:
    a) anagen
    b) catagen
    c) biogen
    d) telogen

    _____

42. The resting phase of hair growth lasts approximately:
    a) 1–2 weeks
    b) 1–2 months
    c) 2–6 years
    d) 2–6 months

    _____

43. About _____% of the hair is in the resting phase at any one time.
    a) 90
    b) 50
    c) 75
    d) 10

    _____

44. Average daily hair loss is approximately:
    a) 40–50 hairs
    b) 400–1,000 hairs
    c) 40–100 hairs
    d) 10–30 hairs

    _____

45. The average head has about _____ individual shafts of hair.
    a) 50,000
    b) 100,000
    c) 1,000,000
    d) 10,000

    _____

46. Redheads have approximately _____ shafts of hair on the head.
    a) 140,000
    b) 19,000
    c) 9,000
    d) 90,000

    _____

47. Hair flowing in the same direction is the:
    a) natural parting
    b) hair stream
    c) circular pattern
    d) main division
    _____

48. A whorl is formed when hair grows in a:
    a) conflicting pattern
    b) circular pattern
    c) curly and straight pattern on one head
    d) tuft pattern
    _____

49. A cowlick is formed when a tuft of hair:
    a) grows to a point
    b) grows in a circle
    c) is standing up
    d) will not curl
    _____

50. One common hair myth is:
    a) hair is shed daily
    b) keratin is protein
    c) the medulla may be absent in fine hair
    d) hair grows after death
    _____

51. The three hair shapes are round, oval, and:
    a) rectangular
    b) almost flat
    c) triangular
    d) half-moon
    _____

52. Straight hair has a/an _____ shape.
    a) round
    b) almost flat
    c) oval
    d) half-moon
    _____

53. The true guide for a hair shape is:
    a) a person's age
    b) a person's nationality
    c) the direction of a hair as it projects out of the follicle
    d) the size of the hair root
    _____

54. A client's hair must be _____ before any service.
    a) shampooed
    b) analyzed
    c) sterilized
    d) thoroughly dried
    _____

55. The only one of the five senses not used when analyzing the hair is:
    a) touch
    b) taste
    c) smell
    d) sight
    _____

56. *Hair texture* refers to the hair's:
    a) ability to absorb moisture
    b) degree of straightness or curliness
    c) ability to hold a full style
    d) degree of coarseness or fineness
    _____

57. _____ hair has the greatest diameter.
    a) Fine
    b) Straight
    c) Gray
    d) Coarse
    _____

58. Wiry hair may have a hard, glassy finish caused by:
    a) raised cuticle scales
    b) flat cuticle scales
    c) overconditioning
    d) age
    _____

59. The hair's ability to absorb moisture is its:
    a) texture
    b) elasticity
    c) porosity
    d) density
    _____

60. Resistant hair is said to have:
    a) good porosity
    b) hygroscopic quality
    c) moderate porosity
    d) poor porosity
    _____

61. Extreme porosity may be caused by:
    a) conditioning treatments
    b) damage from faulty treatments
    c) strand testing
    d) brushing hair before shampooing
    _____

62. The ability of the hair to stretch and return to its original form without breaking is known as:
    a) porosity
    b) density
    c) texture
    d) elasticity
    _____

63. Hair can be stretched 40–50% when:
    a) damaged
    b) dry
    c) wet
    d) permanently waved
    _____

64. It may take a longer amount of time for chemicals to penetrate hair with:
    a) medium texture
    b) good porosity
    c) poor porosity
    d) fine texture
    _____

65. Scientists believe approximately 95% of hair loss is caused by a progressive condition called:
   a) alopecia areata
   b) androgenetic alopecia
   c) chemotherapy
   d) generic alopecia
   _____

66. By age 35, almost _____% of men show some degree of hair loss.
   a) 10
   b) 95
   c) 25
   d) 40
   _____

67. The gene for the most common type of hair loss may be:
   a) altered
   b) inherited from either side of the family or both sides
   c) inherited from the maternal side only
   d) responsible for pityriasis
   _____

68. In men, a horseshoe-shaped fringe of hair is referred to as:
   a) male pattern baldness
   b) fringe pattern baldness
   c) horseshoe baldness
   d) dome baldness
   _____

69. A miniaturization of certain scalp follicles contributes to:
   a) androgenetic alopecia
   b) postpartum alopecia
   c) alopecia areata
   d) telogen effluvium
   _____

70. The hair loss process is a gradual conversion of terminal hair follicles to:
   a) supercilia hair
   b) horseshoe shaped follicles
   c) vellus-like follicles
   d) enlarged follicles
   _____

71. Androgenetic alopecia:
   a) does not change follicle size
   b) does not alter the number of follicles
   c) alters follicle structure
   d) increases follicle numbers
   _____

72. Alopecia areata is defined as:
   a) slow baldness
   b) male pattern baldness
   c) sudden hair loss in round or irregular patches
   d) hair loss due to repetitive traction on the hair due to pulling or twisting
   _____

73. Telogen effluvium:
   a) can be reversed
   b) happens to everyone
   c) is hereditary
   d) is incurable
   _____

74. Excessive application of chemicals or excessive use of hot combs may cause:
    a) alopecia areata
    b) telogen effluvium
    c) androgenetic alopecia
    d) traumatic alopecia   _____

75. Asking questions about a client's family history with hair loss helps identify:
    a) alopecia areata
    b) telogen effluvium
    c) androgenetic alopecia
    d) postpartum alopecia   _____

76. The cosmetologist may recognize miniaturized hairs on a client's scalp by their:
    a) flat ends
    b) round ends
    c) split ends
    d) pointy ends   _____

77. In women, androgenetic alopecia may be recognized by:
    a) a horseshoe shape
    b) a full parting
    c) a smaller diameter ponytail
    d) a fuller diameter ponytail   _____

78. When testing for telogen effluvium, if more than _____ hairs come out easily, the client has active shedding and may be going through telogen effluvium.
    a) 15–20
    b) 3–5
    c) 30–40
    d) 1–3   _____

79. When evaluating hair loss, the time lapse between evaluations should be:
    a) 4–6 weeks
    b) 2–4 weeks
    c) 2–4 months
    d) 4–6 months   _____

80. The degree of hair loss in men can be evaluated by rating:
    a) texture and elasticity
    b) pattern and density
    c) texture and density
    d) pattern and texture   _____

81. In male pattern baldness, the scalp is divided into the front, the mid-area, and the:
    a) apex
    b) parietal
    c) vortex
    d) vertex   _____

82. A topical solution applied to the scalp that is medically proven to regrow hair is:
    a) finasteride
    b) follicidil
    c) monoxidil
    d) methacrylate _____

83. Enlarging miniaturized follicles and reversing the miniaturization process prolongs the growth phase of the hair cycle and:
    a) removes vellus
    b) encourages root formation
    c) allows longer and thicker hair to grow
    d) eliminates postpartum alopecia _____

84. A prescription pill for the treatment of androgenetic alopecia is:
    a) finasteride
    b) follicidil
    c) monoxidil
    d) methacrylate _____

85. The technical term for gray hair is:
    a) mottiltis
    b) monilethrix
    c) canities
    d) ash _____

86. Alternate bands of gray and dark hair is called:
    a) smoky
    b) ringed hair
    c) canities
    d) acquired canities _____

87. The condition characterized by an abnormal development of hair on areas of the body normally bearing only vellus hair is known as:
    a) hypertrichosis
    b) monilethrix
    c) canities
    d) fragilitas crinium _____

88. Trichoptilosis is the technical name for:
    a) burnt hair
    b) split ends
    c) gray hair
    d) ringed hair _____

89. Trichorrhexis nodosa may be identified by:
    a) a horseshoe pattern
    b) brittle hair
    c) lack of elasticity
    d) nodular swellings along the hair shaft _____

90. The technical term for beaded hair is:
    a) trichorrhexis nodosa
    b) nodositis
    c) monilethrix
    d) hirsuties _____

91. Fragilitis crinium is identified by:
    a) knotting
    b) beads or nodes
    c) split ends
    d) brittle hair   _____

92. The medical term for dandruff is:
    a) pityriasis
    b) pediculosis
    c) epithelialitis
    d) monilethrix   _____

93. An itchy scalp with small white scales either attached to the scalp in masses or scattered loosely in the hair is an indication of:
    a) hirsuties
    b) pityriasis capitis simplex
    c) pediculosis
    d) tinea   _____

94. Pityriasis steadoides is also referred to as:
    a) dry dandruff
    b) greasy dandruff
    c) lice
    d) ringworm   _____

95. Tinea is commonly carried by scales or hairs containing:
    a) dandruff
    b) product buildup
    c) lice
    d) fungi   _____

96. The medical term for ringworm is:
    a) pediculosis
    b) tinea
    c) pityriasis
    d) scutula   _____

97. Red papules, or spots, at the opening of the hair follicles are symptoms of:
    a) tinea favosa
    b) pediculosis
    c) tinea capitis
    d) hypertinea   _____

98. Tinea favosa may be identified by:
    a) red papules
    b) white flakes
    c) multiple furuncles
    d) dry, sulfur-yellow,
       cuplike crusts
       on the scalp   _____

99. Scabies is caused by:
    a) spores
    b) the itch mite
    c) tinea
    d) abnormal hair loss   _____

100. Pediculosis is caused by:
a) the itch mite
b) head lice
c) tinea
d) a vegetable parasite _____

101. A furuncle is commonly known as a:
a) wart
b) cold sore
c) follicle infection
d) boil _____

102. A basic requisite for a healthy scalp is cleanliness and:
a) conditioning
b) stimulation
c) tightness
d) dryness _____

103. Scalp massage for a normal scalp should be performed:
a) daily
b) monthly
c) biweekly
d) weekly _____

104. With each massage movement, place the hands:
a) on top of the hair
b) under the hair
c) perpendicular to the head
d) vertical to the head _____

105. Regular scalp treatments may help slow some types of hair loss because of:
a) human contact
b) dry heat
c) increase of blood flow
d) proper rinsing _____

106. When performing a scalp treatment for dry hair and scalp, avoid the use of:
a) emollient materials
b) gentle soaps
c) a natural bristle brush
d) high-alcohol materials _____

107. When performing a scalp treatment for oily hair and scalp, sebum should be:
a) dried on the scalp
b) removed with high-frequency current and an alcohol tonic
c) removed with the correct degree of pressing or squeezing
d) brushed away _____

108. The product commonly used for dry hair treatments contains:
a) monoxidil
b) astringent
c) phenol
d) cholesterol _____

109. Applying heat when using a conditioning treatment acts to:
    a) close the cuticle
    b) open the cuticle
    c) close the cortex
    d) force conditioner into the medulla
    _____

110. Hair treatments may be given a week or 10 days before a chemical service or:
    a) the day after a chemical service
    b) the day of a chemical service
    c) 2 weeks after a chemical service
    d) a week or 10 days after a chemical service
    _____

Draping

1. Proper draping serves to protect the client's skin and:
   - a) jewelry
   - b) clothing
   - c) hairline
   - d) nape area _____

2. Methods of draping may vary depending on:
   - a) the client's neck size
   - b) the service performed
   - c) the cosmetologist's preference
   - d) the draping materials available _____

3. Before draping, the cosmetologist must:
   - a) wear rubber gloves
   - b) adjust the towel
   - c) sanitize hands
   - d) section the hair _____

4. A neck strip or towel is necessary to prevent the client's skin from:
   - a) touching the cape
   - b) feeling uncomfortable
   - c) getting wet
   - d) chemical contact _____

5. Possible skin irritation from chemicals is prevented by proper draping with a cape and:
   - a) a plastic cap
   - b) a neck strip
   - c) a terrycloth towel
   - d) absorbent pads _____

6. Every effort must be made to prevent the cape from touching the client's skin because it could be:
   - a) cold to the skin
   - b) a carrier of disease
   - c) slightly damp
   - d) irritating _____

7. A neck strip may be used when draping for a haircut to allow:
    a) cutting on the skin
    b) the hair to fall naturally
    c) the cape to close snugly
    d) the client to remain cooler   _____

8. Before draping, clients should:
    a) remove their jewelry
    b) wash their hands
    c) brush their hair
    d) request a draping method   _____

9. Draping for a comb-out should include:
    a) a towel at the neck
    b) a shampoo cape
    c) two towels around the neck
    d) a neck strip under the cape   _____

10. Improper draping places your client's comfort and _____ in jeopardy.
    a) trust
    b) faith
    c) respect
    d) safety   _____

Shampooing, Rinsing, and Conditioning

1. The main purpose of shampoos is to:
   a) make hair easier to style
   b) cleanse the hair and scalp
   c) disinfect the hair and scalp
   d) make the hair and scalp smell better _____

2. Before applying the shampoo, wet the hair with:
   a) cold water
   b) hot water
   c) warm water
   d) a strong spray of water _____

3. Strong alkaline shampoos make hair:
   a) soft
   b) dry
   c) shed easily
   d) contract _____

4. Combing hair after a shampoo should begin:
   a) at the nape
   b) at either side
   c) in the bang area
   d) in the crown _____

5. After a regular shampoo, rinse with:
   a) cold water
   b) a soft mist
   c) hot water
   d) a strong spray _____

6. Thorough brushing of the scalp and hair should NOT be done before a:
   a) shampoo
   b) haircolor
   c) haircut
   d) scalp treatment _____

7. What should be used when massaging and lathering the client's scalp and hair during a shampoo?
   a) the thumbs only
   b) rubber gloves
   c) the palm of the hand
   d) the cushions of your fingers _____

8. During rinsing, one finger should be over the edge of the spray nozzle in order to:
   a) monitor the water temperature
   b) keep the client's hair out
   c) determine the water spray pattern
   d) hold the nozzle in place _____

9. The term pH stands for:
   a) potential hydrogen
   b) parts of hydrogen
   c) possible humidity
   d) phosphorus and hydrogen _____

10. Medicated shampoos will affect:
    a) the style results
    b) the color of tinted hair
    c) cuticle size
    d) the conditioner process _____

11. Do not give a dry shampoo before:
    a) styling
    b) braiding
    c) cutting
    d) a chemical treatment _____

12. Brittle or dry hair should be cleansed with a/an:
    a) alkaline shampoo
    b) cream shampoo
    c) acid-balanced shampoo
    d) dry shampoo _____

13. If used too frequently, conditioners may:
    a) improve hair health
    b) form a buildup on hair
    c) improve scalp health
    d) affect hair growth _____

14. The type of hairbrush recommended for use before a shampoo is:
    a) plastic bristle
    b) natural bristle
    c) nylon bristle
    d) rubber bristle _____

15. Brushing should be performed before a shampoo because it:
    a) allows time for consultation
    b) is soothing to the client
    c) stimulates blood circulation
    d) decreases static _____

16. Acid rinses are given to:
    a) remove soap scum
    b) add color to the hair
    c) remove yellow streaks from gray hair
    d) open the cuticle layer _____

17. To make hair slick and smooth, use a:
    a) cream rinse
    c) dry shampoo
    b) medicated shampoo
    d) styling gel _____

18. A rinse that helps close and harden the cuticle imbrications after a tint or toner application is a/an:
    a) acid-balanced rinse
    c) henna rinse
    b) alkaline rinse
    d) temporary color rinse _____

19. Hair rinses consist of a mixture of water, coloring agent, and:
    a) an alkaline
    c) an oil
    b) an acid
    d) henna _____

20. Citric acid is obtained from:
    a) lactose
    c) vinegar
    b) vegetables
    d) lime, orange, or lemon juice _____

21. A shampoo that has a pH of 5.5 is considered to be:
    a) neutral
    c) alkaline
    b) harsh
    d) acid _____

22. Minor dandruff conditions may be controlled by:
    a) plain water rinses
    c) citric acid rinses
    b) medicated shampoos
    d) acid shampoo _____

23. Proper shampooing helps prevent:
    a) scalp disorders
    c) split ends
    b) dry hair
    d) static _____

24. Medicated rinses help control:
    a) color fading
    c) hair thinning
    b) tangles
    d) dandruff _____

25. Hard water may not allow a shampoo to lather because it contains:
    a) anti-lather ingredients
    c) minerals
    b) chemicals
    d) sodium hypochlorite _____

Haircutting

1. When selecting a suitable hairstyle for a client you must consider:
   a) the implement used
   b) the hair texture
   c) current fashions
   d) the client's wardrobe _____

2. Partings for haircutting are usually:
   a) 1/4"
   b) 1"
   c) 1/2"
   d) 1/8" _____

3. If you cut past your second knuckle, the amount of _____ changes and causes an uneven haircut.
   a) continuity
   b) resistance
   c) tension
   d) pressure _____

4. Beveling is performed by:
   a) cutting the hair straight across
   b) slithering
   c) cutting with the points of the shears
   d) holding the shears at an angle other than 90 degrees _____

5. Blunt cutting involves:
   a) cutting the hair straight across
   b) effilating
   c) thinning
   d) holding the shears at an angle other than 90 degrees _____

6. An elevation is:
   a) cutting the hair straight across
   b) another term for layering
   c) the angle the hair is lifted from the head
   d) another term for graduation _____

7. A graduation is:
   a) another term for layering
   b) a stacked exterior area
   c) how far the hair is lifted
   d) another term for elevation _____

8. The section of hair that determines the length of the cut is the:
   a) parting
   b) guideline
   c) section
   d) graduation line _____

9. When hair falls naturally and each subsection is slightly shorter than the guide, it is known as:
   a) blunt cutting
   b) undercutting
   c) notching or pointing
   d) layering _____

10. Cutting with the points of the shear to create texture in the hair ends is known as:
    a) blunt cutting
    b) undercutting
    c) notching
    d) layering _____

11. Cutting the hair so each parting is slightly longer than the previous parting to encourage hair to curl under is known as:
    a) blunt cutting
    b) undercutting
    c) notching or pointing
    d) shingling _____

12. Weight is the area in a haircut where:
    a) the least amount of hair falls
    b) the hair curls under
    c) the largest amount of hair falls
    d) the most texture is present _____

13. A razor shaper cuts hair with a _____ edge than the shear.
    a) softer
    b) more defined
    c) sharper
    d) cleaner _____

14. Thinning shears are used to:
    a) add volume
    b) create short tapers quickly
    c) remove bulk
    d) taper hair ends _____

15. Removing superfluous hair and creating clean lines around the perimeter of a haircut is best accomplished with:
    a) clippers
    b) a depilatory
    c) a straight razor
    d) an edger _____

16. The amount of elevation from the head form is measured in:
    a) degrees
    c) subsections
    b) partings
    d) inches   _____

17. Parallel lines:
    a) are in between horizontal   c) intersect at 90 degrees
       and vertical
    b) never meet .   d) are not used in haircutting   _____

18. Perpendicular lines:
    a) are in between horizontal   c) intersect at 90 degrees
       and vertical
    b) never meet   d) involve using thinning shears _____

19. The lines used for blending and special design haircuts are:
    a) perpendicular
    c) parallel
    b) diagonal
    d) horizontal   _____

20. The lines used in low-elevation haircuts are:
    a) perpendicular
    c) vertical
    b) diagonal
    d) horizontal   _____

21. Maintaining control over the point of the shears while combing
    the hair during a haircut is accomplished by:
    a) bracing the shears   c) knuckling the shears
    b) palming the shears   d) keeping the thumb
                                         in the shears   _____

22. _____ hair cannot be controlled when cut too short.
    a) Fine   c) Medium-textured
    b) Coarse   d) Straight   _____

23. Leave extra length in a haircut for cowlicks and:
    a) nape hair
    c) whorls
    b) sideburns
    d) crown   _____

24. Dividing the hair for a haircut is known as:
    a) sectioning
    c) preparation
    b) parting
    d) shaping   _____

25. A guide in a haircut that does not move is:
    a) an interior guide
    b) stationary
    c) traveling
    d) an exterior guide _____

26. A 90-degree elevation is a:
    a) low elevation
    b) reverse elevation
    c) high elevation
    d) blended elevation _____

27. A one-length haircut is best achieved using a:
    a) zero-degree elevation
    b) 180-degree elevation
    c) 90-degree elevation
    d) blended elevation _____

28. Scissors-over-comb is used to:
    a) create volume
    b) correct cowlicks
    c) create very short tapers
    d) leave length at the nape _____

29. Two places where thinning is not advisable are the:
    a) hairline and nape
    b) part and nape
    c) hairline and part
    d) interior and exterior _____

30. Thinning hair with the shears is known as slithering to:
    a) shearing
    b) effilating
    c) razoring
    d) regulating _____

31. When cutting the hair with a razor, you must hold the hair:
    a) higher than with shears
    b) with your knuckles facing the head
    c) with your palm facing up
    d) with your knuckles facing you _____

32. Using short strokes with the razor will:
    a) remove length
    b) dull the blade
    c) maintain length
    d) take longer _____

33. When using the clippers, you should begin:
    a) at the front hairline
    b) in the crown
    c) at the sides
    d) at the nape _____

34. Slide cutting can be used for:
    a) blending short tapers
    b) removing length
    c) an undercut style
    d) removing superfluous hair _____

35. Scissors-over-comb may be used to:
    a) blend a short crown
    b) blend a short nape with a long crown
    c) blend long nape layers
    d) blend long bangs with a short crown

    _____

36. The results of a high-elevation haircut should be:
    a) longer in the crown
    b) longer in the nape
    c) the same length throughout the head
    d) various blended lengths

    _____

37. If the head is pushed forward during the haircut, the results will be:
    a) graduated ends
    b) longer underneath
    c) wispy
    d) undercut

    _____

38. Bangs may be sectioned with a curved section or:
    a) triangular
    b) rectangular
    c) oval
    d) square

    _____

39. The number of degrees in a full circle is:
    a) 45
    b) 180
    c) 90
    d) 360

    _____

40. Hair must be _____ when cutting.
    a) saturated
    b) uniformly wet or dry
    c) dry
    d) partially wet

    _____

Artistry in Hairstyling

1. The five elements of design are form, space, line, texture, and:
   - a) volume
   - b) color
   - c) silhouette
   - d) appearance

   _____

2. The area a hairstyle occupies inside the form refers to its:
   - a) line
   - b) silhouette
   - c) texture
   - d) space

   _____

3. Space is three-dimensional. It has length, width, and:
   - a) lines
   - b) color
   - c) depth
   - d) texture

   _____

4. Line creates the form, design, and_____ of a hairstyle.
   - a) volume
   - b) depth
   - c) space
   - d) movement

   _____

5. The four basic types of style lines are horizontal, vertical, diagonal, and:
   - a) curved
   - b) perpendicular
   - c) parallel
   - d) flat

   _____

6. A horizontal line creates:
   - a) a narrow illusion
   - b) waves
   - c) width
   - d) height

   _____

7. Curved lines repeating in opposite directions are:
   - a) curls
   - b) waves
   - c) used to create clash
   - d) used to decrease volume

   _____

8. An example of a single line design is a:
   a) finger wave
   b) one-length hairstyle
   c) layered look
   d) blended horizontal and vertical style   _____

9. Contrasting lines are reserved for clients with the _____ to carry off a strong look.
   a) complexion
   b) wardrobe
   c) personality
   d) spouse   _____

10. Transitional lines are usually:
    a) curved
    b) horizontal
    c) vertical
    d) diagonal   _____

11. The illusion of _____ is created by alternating warm and cool or light and dark colors.
    a) youth
    b) volume
    c) depth
    d) texture   _____

12. When light and dark colors are used together, the darker hair seems to:
    a) appear closer to the surface
    b) recede below the surface
    c) fade
    d) brighten   _____

13. Light or warm colors in the top or bang area create:
    a) width
    b) interest
    c) texture
    d) length   _____

14. In order to reflect the most light, straight hair is usually cut and styled:
    a) in one length
    b) in contrasting lines
    c) in many layers
    d) with a variety of angles   _____

15. The actual surface quality of the hair is referred to as:
    a) density
    b) texture
    c) volume
    d) depth   _____

16. The maximum number of different textures to use in a design is:
    a) 2
    b) 4
    c) 3
    d) 5   _____

17. Use curly textures to:
    a) accent the face
    b) elongate the neck
    c) narrow a round head shape
    d) soften square or rectangular features _____

18. The five art principles important for hair design are proportion, balance, rhythm, emphasis, and:
    a) texture
    b) harmony
    c) color
    d) symmetry _____

19. The ideal ratio for hairstyle design is either 3 parts face to 2 parts hair or:
    a) 3 parts face to 3 parts hair
    b) 2 parts face to 3 parts hair
    c) 2 parts face to 2 parts hair
    d) 1 part face to 1 part hair _____

20. The proportion of 3 parts face to 2 parts hair is used when the client:
    a) wants attention to the face
    b) wants to minimize features
    c) has poor skin
    d) wants to draw attention away from the face _____

21. To measure symmetry, divide the face into:
    a) two equal sides
    b) three proportions
    c) top and bottom
    d) four equal parts _____

22. Opposite sides of the hairstyle are a different length or volume if the design is:
    a) asymmetrical
    b) out of proportion
    c) symmetrical
    d) in style _____

23. An example of a fast rhythm pattern is:
    a) larger shapings
    b) one-length styles
    c) long waves
    d) tight curls _____

24. When the design starts out with a large pattern that changes to a smaller one, it is called:
    a) horizontal rhythm
    b) increasing rhythm
    c) decreasing rhythm
    d) alternating rhythm _____

25. A boring hairstyle is sometimes created when _____ is used.
    a) decreasing rhythm
    b) alternating rhythm
    c) increasing rhythm
    d) only one rhythm _____

26. The place the eye sees first in a hairstyle is called the point of:
    a) proportion
    c) emphasis
    b) harmony
    d) balance
    _____

27. The most important of the art principles is:
    a) proportion
    c) emphasis
    b) harmony
    d) balance
    _____

28. If a client has a narrow forehead and wide jaw and chin line (or a pear-shaped face), the aim is to:
    a) reduce forehead width
    c) increase jaw width
    b) create the illusion of length
    d) create the illusion of width in the forehead
    _____

29. The basic hair parting for bangs is:
    a) oblong
    c) triangular
    b) diagonal
    d) square
    _____

30. The middle third of the face consists of the eyes and:
    a) nose
    c) jaw
    b) lips
    d) forehead
    _____

31. The square facial type can be identified by the square jawline and:
    a) round hairline
    c) narrow forehead
    b) hollow cheeks
    d) straight hairline
    _____

32. The most flattering style for the pear-shaped face includes:
    a) the crown styled flat
    c) no hair on the face
    b) height
    d) wispy hair at the nape
    _____

33. A narrow forehead may be made to look wider using highlights at the:
    a) nape
    c) temples
    b) crown
    d) parting
    _____

34. The convex profile, receding forehead, and large forehead may all be styled:
    a) with bangs
    c) with a lot of volume
    b) away from the face
    d) fuller at the nape
    _____

35. The hair parting used to make thin hair appear fuller is the:
    a) zigzag
    b) center
    c) diagonal
    d) side

_____

Wet Hairstyling

1. A good waving lotion is harmless to the hair and:
   a) dries on contact
   b) does not flake when dry
   c) leaves a mild residue
   d) should be used liberally _____

2. Finger wave lotion should be applied:
   a) to one side of the head at a time
   b) to the entire head after shampooing
   c) with a brush
   d) while wearing gloves _____

3. Pinching or pushing ridges with fingers will create:
   a) underdirection of the ridge
   b) splits
   c) overdirection of the ridge
   d) inconsistent waves _____

4. With a side-part hairstyle, the finger wave should start:
   a) on the left side
   b) on the heavy side
   c) on the right side
   d) on the light side _____

5. The term *shadow wave* indicates a hairstyle with:
   a) high ridges
   b) clash
   c) low ridges
   d) deep waves _____

6. The three main parts of a pin curl are the base, stem, and:
   a) curl
   b) wave
   c) medulla
   d) circle _____

7. The stationary part of the pin curl is the:
   a) curl
   b) stem
   c) circle
   d) base _____

8. The section of the pin curl between the base and the first arc is the:
   a) circle
   b) stem
   c) wave
   d) curl _____

9. A tight, firm, long-lasting curl is produced by the:
   a) full-stem curl
   b) no-stem curl
   c) half-stem curl
   d) mobile stem curl _____

10. The greatest curl mobility is achieved with the:
    a) full-stem curl
    b) no-stem curl
    c) half-stem curl
    d) 1/4-turn curl _____

11. Open center curls produce:
    a) uniform curls
    b) volume
    c) waves that decrease in size
    d) curls that decrease in size _____

12. When a fluffy curl is desired, use:
    a) open center curls
    b) forward movement curls
    c) closed center curls
    d) reverse movement curls _____

13. Curls formed in the same direction as the movement of the hands of a clock are:
    a) counterclockwise curls
    b) 8:00 curls
    c) stem directed curls
    d) clockwise curls _____

14. A section of hair that is molded into a design and serves as the base for a curl or wave pattern is a:
    a) parting
    b) shaping
    c) section
    d) base _____

15. Always begin pin curls at the _____ end of a shaping.
    a) open
    b) bottom
    c) top
    d) circular _____

16. The most commonly used bases for pin curls are rectangular, triangular, square, and:
    a) flat
    b) arc
    c) cascade
    d) oblong _____

17. A finished curl is not affected by the:
    a) size of the curl
    b) shape of the base
    c) amount of hair used
    d) direction of curl   _____

18. Triangular bases are used:
    a) to avoid tangling
    b) to add height
    c) to avoid splits in the finished style
    d) to maintain a smooth upsweep look   _____

19. Pin curl bases that are used for curly hairstyles without much volume or lift are:
    a) rectangular
    b) arc
    c) triangular
    d) square   _____

20. Curls sliced out of a shaping are known as:
    a) ribbon curls
    b) carved curls
    c) cascade curls
    d) barrel curls   _____

21. The shaping that allows a wave to remain the same width throughout the shaping is the:
    a) circular shaping
    b) oblong shaping
    c) forward shaping
    d) oval shaping   _____

22. Pin curls are correctly anchored when they:
    a) have closed centers
    b) cover the circle
    c) start at the open end
    d) require two clips   _____

23. Curls used to create a wave behind a ridge are called:
    a) brush waves
    b) shadow curls
    c) skip waves
    d) ridge curls   _____

24. Two rows of ridge curls create:
    a) a strong wave pattern
    b) height
    c) soft curls
    d) a crested wave curl   _____

25. When some height is need during the transition from stand-up pin curls to sculptured curls, use:
    a) brush waves
    b) semi-stand-up curls
    c) cascade curls
    d) lazy curls   _____

26. Barrel curls are large stand-up pin curls on a:
    a) triangular base
    b) oblong base
    c) arc base
    d) rectangular base
    _____

27. A roller holds the equivalent of:
    a) 5 stand-up curls
    b) 2–4 stand-up curls
    c) 1 stand-up curl
    d) 1/2 of a stand-up curl
    _____

28. The size of the curl in a roller set is determined by the:
    a) size of the base
    b) direction of the curl
    c) setting pattern
    d) size of the roller
    _____

29. Volume is determined by the size of the roller and:
    a) number of rollers used
    b) the direction of the curl
    c) how it sits on its base
    d) anchoring clips used
    _____

30. An on-base curl produces:
    a) medium volume
    b) full volume
    c) the least amount of volume
    d) a crisp curl
    _____

31. For the least amount of volume in a roller set use the:
    a) on-base method
    b) one-half-base method
    c) off-base method
    d) open-end method
    _____

32. An indentation roller is usually placed:
    a) in front of a volume roller
    b) vertical to a volume roller
    c) horizontal to a volume roller
    d) behind a volume roller
    _____

33. If hair is wound 1 1/2 turns around a roller, it will create:
    a) a C-shape
    b) a wave
    c) an explosion of curl
    d) a well-anchored curl
    _____

34. A C-shape will result if the hair is wound:
    a) 2 1/2 turns around the roller
    b) 1 complete turn around the roller
    c) 5 turns around the roller
    d) 1 1/2 turns around the roller
    _____

35. A stronger curvature movement may be achieved by using:
    a) cylinder rollers
    b) blue rollers
    c) tapered rollers
    d) Velcro rollers
    _____

36. When a smooth comb-out is desired, be sure to:
   a) use a pick
   b) brush the hair smooth
   c) use a wide-tooth comb
   d) brush hair ends only   _____

37. Most failures in combing out hairstyles are due primarily to:
   a) the client's hair
   b) choice of setting gel
   c) improperly set hair
   d) smoothing too much   _____

38. Back-comb areas that require:
   a) no height
   b) volume
   c) less fullness
   d) emphasis   _____

39. *Teasing, ratting, matting,* and *French lacing* are other terms for:
   a) smoothing
   b) back-combing
   c) back-brushing
   d) comb-outs   _____

40. *Ruffing* is another name for:
   a) smoothing
   b) back-combing
   c) back-brushing
   d) relaxing the set   _____

41. Two types of French braids are the invisible and:
   a) 2 strand
   b) overlapped
   c) inverted
   d) regular   _____

42. Cornrowing is done in the same fashion as:
   a) visible French braids
   b) overlapped braids
   c) invisible French braids
   d) regular braids   _____

Thermal Hairstyling

1. For white, lightened, or tinted hair, it is advisable to use thermal irons that:
   a) are large in diameter
   b) are lukewarm
   c) have a built-in thermostat
   d) contain less steel   _____

2. Electric vaporizing irons should not be used on pressed hair because they cause the hair to:
   a) revert
   b) break
   c) straighten
   d) flatten   _____

3. Overheated irons are often ruined because the metal loses its:
   a) color
   b) balance
   c) temper
   d) shape   _____

4. A conventional thermal iron is:
   a) electric self-heated
   b) stove heated
   c) electric self-heated, vaporizing
   d) coal heated   _____

5. The required temperature of heated thermal irons depends on the:
   a) type of irons selected
   b) texture of the hair
   c) cosmetologist's speed
   d) size of the heater   _____

6. The technique of drying and styling damp hair in one operation is called:
   a) croquignole styling
   b) thermal iron styling
   c) thermal styling
   d) blow-dry styling   _____

7. To hold an even temperature, thermal irons should be made of the best quality:
   a) hard rubber
   b) zinc
   c) steel
   d) magnesium   _____

8. The temperature of heated thermal irons is tested on:
   a) a strand of hair
   b) a piece of tissue paper
   c) a damp cloth
   d) wax paper _____

9. The art of creating curls with the aid of heated irons and a comb is known as:
   a) hot setting
   b) spiral curling
   c) thermal curling
   d) swivel curling _____

10. The thermal iron curl that provides maximum lift is the:
    a) off-base curl
    b) volume-base curl
    c) half-base curl
    d) full-base curl _____

11. Setting and drying the hair with the use of electric comb and styling comb is called:
    a) Marcel waving
    b) thermal waving
    c) French waving
    d) air waving _____

12. A thermal comb should be made of:
    a) plastic
    b) hard rubber
    c) steel
    d) wood _____

13. To give a finished appearance to hair ends, use:
    a) end curls
    b) spiral curls
    c) the figure 8 technique
    d) the figure 6 technique _____

14. To ensure a good thermal curl or wave, the hair must be:
    a) well oiled
    b) damp
    c) clean
    d) warm from the blow dryer _____

15. The styling portion of a thermal iron consists of a rod and:
    a) prong
    b) cord
    c) shell
    d) swivel _____

16. Volume thermal iron curls are created to provide the finished hairstyle with:
    a) depth
    b) indentation
    c) lift
    d) tension _____

17. Before hair is combed out after blow-dry styling, it should be thoroughly:
    a) ruffed
    b) cooled
    c) teased
    d) heated
    _____

18. Before using the blow dryer, be sure the:
    a) diffuser is attached
    b) styling brushes are warm
    c) air intake is clean
    d) hair is sectioned
    _____

19. Fishhook hair ends are caused when the:
    a) irons are too hot
    b) curl is started too low
    c) curl is started too high
    d) hair ends protrude from the irons
    _____

20. An electrical device especially designed for drying and styling the hair in a single operation is a:
    a) thermal dryer
    b) hood dryer
    c) blow dryer
    d) curl dryer
    _____

21. For successful blow-dry styling, the air should be directed from the scalp area to:
    a) the floor
    b) the hair ends
    c) the face
    d) the root area
    _____

22. In order to assure complete dryness of the hair, the blower is used in a:
    a) back and forth movement
    b) front to back pattern
    c) vertical motion
    d) stop and go movement
    _____

23. A blow-dry style will not hold if:
    a) the hair is straight
    b) the hair is curly
    c) styling products are used
    d) the scalp is damp
    _____

24. Excessive blow-drying may cause dryness and:
    a) deep waves
    b) split ends
    c) stunted hair growth
    d) shadow waves
    _____

25. An air waver comb may be used with a:
    a) round brush
    b) steamer
    c) metal comb
    d) vapor oil
    _____

26. The principal cosmetics used in blow-dry styling are hair and scalp conditioners, hair sprays, and:
   a) acid rinses
   b) surfactants
   c) styling lotions
   d) water
   _____

27. Another term for thermal waving is:
   a) Grateau waving
   b) pressing
   c) ironing
   d) Marcel waving
   _____

28. The client's scalp is protected from burns during a thermal iron styling by using:
   a) petroleum jelly
   b) the smallest diameter iron
   c) the iron on damp hair
   d) a hard rubber comb
   _____

29. The styling of hair with an air waver is performed in the same manner as:
   a) thermal waving
   b) blow-out waving
   c) chemical waving
   d) finger waving
   _____

30. Blow-dry styling may be performed with a brush or:
   a) crimper
   b) comb
   c) rollers
   d) curling iron
   _____

Permanent Waving

1. Vigorously brushing the hair before a permanent wave may cause:
   a) hair discoloration
   b) scalp tightening
   c) healthy hair to fall out
   d) scalp irritations _____

2. Before a permanent wave, a mild shampoo should be accompanied by:
   a) gentle scalp manipulations
   b) kneading scalp manipulations
   c) vibratory scalp manipulations
   d) stimulating scalp manipulations _____

3. Before starting a permanent wave, the hair is shampooed and:
   a) thoroughly dried
   b) brushed
   c) towel-dried
   d) the scalp is stimulated _____

4. For a successful permanent wave, it is necessary to have the hair properly:
   a) styled
   b) cut
   c) presoftened
   d) ruffed _____

5. Before perming, hair should be tested for porosity and:
   a) style
   b) elasticity
   c) cut
   d) natural color _____

6. A method of wrapping a permanent wave that is suitable for extra long hair is the:
   a) piggyback method
   b) double halo method
   c) dropped crown method
   d) single halo method _____

7. The proper way to wind the hair for a permanent wave is to:
   a) place the hair in the center of the rod and stretch it in winding
   b) place the hair in the center of the rod and wind it without stretching
   c) distribute hair evenly on the rod and stretch it in winding
   d) distribute hair evenly on rod and wind it smoothly and without stretching
   _____

8. In permanent waving, a longer processing time is usually required for hair that is:
   a) lightened
   b) tinted
   c) porous
   d) resistant
   _____

9. Special perming prewrapping lotions are designed to:
   a) equalize the hair's porosity
   b) accelerate processing
   c) be used on clients with canities
   d) close the cuticle layer
   _____

10. The main active ingredient in acid-balance waving lotions is:
    a) ammonium thioglycolate
    b) glyceryl monothioglycolate
    c) sodium hydroxide
    d) hydrogen peroxide
    _____

11. If the fastening band is twisted or stretched too tightly on permanent waving rods, it may cause:
    a) a frizzy curl
    b) straight ends
    c) hair breakage
    d) a longer processing time
    _____

12. In order to determine in advance how the client's hair will react to the permanent waving process, give:
    a) a predisposition test
    b) saturation tests
    c) a mock wave
    d) a test curl
    _____

13. End papers used in wrapping hair ends for a permanent wave must be:
    a) nonporous
    b) waterproof
    c) porous
    d) pre-folded
    _____

14. Cold waving lotion:
    a) hardens hair
    b) softens hair
    c) sets hair
    d) closes the cuticle
    _____

15. A benefit derived from using an alkaline perm is:
    a) a softer curl
    b) that it is made for delicate hair
    c) a slower processing time
    d) a strong curl pattern _____

16. Always check manufacturer's directions to see if _____
    is needed.
    a) a plastic cap
    b) shampooing
    c) a neutralizer
    d) a specialty wrap _____

17. Choosing the appropriate perm must be done:
    a) by the client
    b) after careful analysis
    c) according to price
    d) before the consultation _____

18. Ninety percent of the hair's total weight is due to the:
    a) cuticle
    b) number of disulfide bonds present
    c) cortex
    d) amount of melanin present _____

19. A shorter processing time in permanent waving is usually
    required for hair that is:
    a) lightened
    b) resistant
    c) wiry
    d) coarse _____

20. The size of the curl or wave in permanent waving is controlled
    by the:
    a) size of the perm rod
    b) cold wave solution
    c) processing time
    d) neutralizer _____

21. Overprocessing in permanent waving usually produces:
    a) loose curls
    b) firm curls
    c) frizzy curls
    d) tight curls _____

22. Hair that readily absorbs a permanent waving solution is best
    described as being:
    a) elastic
    b) less dense
    c) medium textured
    d) porous _____

23. When heat is created chemically within the perm product, it is
    known as:
    a) exothermic
    b) endocronic
    c) endothermic
    d) internal processing _____

24. The diameter of the individual hair and its degree of coarseness or fineness are its:
    a) density
    b) texture
    c) porosity
    d) elasticity
    _____

25. The process time for any permanent wave depends on the hair texture and its:
    a) length
    b) porosity
    c) growth pattern
    d) current amount of curl
    _____

26. One reason for success in permanent waving is due to:
    a) the use of concave rods
    b) the use of a tail comb
    c) complete saturation of the hair with waving lotion
    d) draping with towels
    _____

27. Permanent waving combines manual skills and a:
    a) sectioning process
    b) blocking process
    c) chemical process
    d) synthetic process
    _____

28. Average permanent wave partings should match:
    a) the size of the end papers
    b) the size of the desired curl
    c) from crown to nape
    d) the size of the rod
    _____

29. When checking for an "S" pattern, the hair must be unwound:
    a) 2 1/2 turns
    b) 2 full turns
    c) 1 turn
    d) 1 1/2 turns
    _____

30. An important step after rinsing permanent wave lotion from the hair is:
    a) conditioning
    b) blotting
    c) the test curl
    d) removing the rods
    _____

31. In permanent waving, hair that is too curly when wet and frizzy when dry indicates that:
    a) it was underprocessed
    b) it was overprocessed
    c) too much lotion was used
    d) too much neutralizer was used
    _____

32. Hair may darken or break if a permanent wave lotion is applied to hair previously treated with:
    a) paraphenelydiamine
    b) an aniline tint
    c) a metallic tint
    d) sulfonated oils
    _____

33. Winding the hair smoothly and without stretching around the permanent wave rods allows the hair to:
    a) wrap around the rod more times
    b) absorb more water
    c) set during processing
    d) expand during processing
    _____

34. If a permanent wave lotion accidentally drips on the skin, the cosmetologist should immediately apply:
    a) water
    b) a dry towel
    c) neutralizer
    d) more lotion
    _____

35. The use of porous end papers helps to eliminate the possibility of:
    a) overprocessing
    b) using too much tension
    c) fishhooks
    d) underprocessing
    _____

36. The wrapping technique that involves winding the hair from the ends toward the scalp is known as:
    a) croquignole wrapping
    b) the Nessler method
    c) spiral wrapping
    d) flat wrapping
    _____

37. A very mild strength waving solution should be recommended for:
    a) oily hair
    b) tinted hair
    c) coarse hair
    d) virgin hair
    _____

38. Greater curl in the nape area may be achieved with the:
    a) piggyback method
    b) halo wrap method
    c) spiral method
    d) stack method
    _____

39. Correct wrapping in permanent waving permits better:
    a) condensation
    b) circulation
    c) analysis
    d) saturation
    _____

40. The ability of hair to absorb liquids is its:
    a) porosity
    b) texture
    c) elasticity
    d) density
    _____

41. A weak or limp wave formation is the result of:
   a) improper blotting
   b) underprocessing
   c) tension winding
   d) incorrect blocking _____

42. The pH of wave solutions made with ammonium thioglycolate is usually:
   a) alkaline
   b) used for a soft wave pattern
   c) acid
   d) used only with machines _____

43. Protect the client's face and neck during processing with:
   a) petroleum lotion
   b) a vinyl cape
   c) a neck strip
   d) a towel _____

44. Acid-balanced permanent wave solutions have a pH range of:
   a) 8.3–9.4
   b) 7.9–8.4
   c) 4.5–6.5
   d) 7.0–8.5 _____

45. In acid-balanced permanent waving, damage to hair or skin is minimized because:
   a) a neutralizer is required
   b) harsh alkalis are not used
   c) concentrated heat is used
   d) a test curl is required _____

46. Acid-balanced permanent wave solutions are activated by the application of:
   a) a neutralizer
   b) heat
   c) stabilizer
   d) water _____

47. When a perm is activated by outside heat, such as a hooded hair dryer, it is:
   a) endocronic
   b) external processing
   c) exothermic
   d) endothermic _____

48. The ability of hair to stretch and return is its:
   a) porosity
   b) texture
   c) elasticity
   d) density _____

49. To allow the perming process to occur, the _____ bonds must be broken.
   a) disulfide
   b) hydrogen
   c) salt
   d) keratin _____

50. The difference between a body wave and a perm is:
    a) the type of client
    b) the size of the rod used
    c) the solution used
    d) the amount of neutralizer used _____

51. Hair that has been tinted with an ultralight shade or higher than 20 volume peroxide should be treated:
    a) as resistant
    b) as bleached hair
    c) like virgin hair
    d) with a color filler _____

52. Acid-balanced and neutral permanent wave lotions produce:
    a) tight waves
    b) spiral curls
    c) soft, natural-looking waves
    d) shorter-lasting waves _____

Haircoloring

1. The pigment that creates haircolor is:
   a) found in the cuticle
   b) a form of keratin
   c) found in the cortex
   d) predetermined by race _____

2. Quinones are:
   a) colorless
   b) yellow
   c) a copper-protein compound
   d) a purple compound _____

3. Melanocytes:
   a) produce dopa
   b) oxidize into a polymer
   c) distribute melanin
   d) attract protein _____

4. Oxidized tyrosine is known as:
   a) dopachrome
   b) melanosomes
   c) indol-quinone
   d) dopa _____

5. Hair color warmth may be identified by:
   a) eyebrow color
   b) hair color level
   c) eye color
   d) hair texture _____

6. Fine-textured hair:
   a) is resistant to lightening
   b) may process darker when depositing color
   c) has an average response to color
   d) may process lighter when depositing color _____

7. Coarse-textured hair:
   a) may be resistant when lightening
   b) has pigment grouped tightly together
   c) requires the use of a mild lightener
   d) requires a higher volume of peroxide _____

8. When coloring long hair, it is important to consider different:
   a) textures
   b) diameters
   c) lengths of hair
   d) degrees of porosity _____

9. Before applying haircolor, you must identify the client's natural level, tone, and:
   a) wave pattern
   b) age
   c) intensity
   d) hair length _____

10. Levels 1, 2, and 3 are found in approximately _____ of the population.
    a) 5% or less
    b) 15%
    c) 9%
    d) 75% _____

11. The warmth or coolness of a color is known as its:
    a) level
    b) intensity
    c) tone
    d) depth _____

12. Clients with golden skin tones look best in:
    a) warm colors
    b) dark colors
    c) cool colors
    d) neutral colors _____

13. A consultation should be conducted in an area that is:
    a) quiet and lit with fluorescent lights
    b) also a changing area
    c) lit with incandescent lights
    d) well lit and private _____

14. Reflective listening during a consultation is performed by:
    a) pausing after the client answers
    b) repeating what the client has said
    c) asking questions twice
    d) allowing the client to speak without asking a lot of questions _____

15. Medication, vitamins, and _____ can affect haircolor results.
    a) personal grooming budget
    b) drinking water
    c) the amount of time the client spends on their hair
    d) home hair care products _____

16. It is important to explain to your client before applying color:
    a) the time and monetary investment involved
    b) the difference between various brands
    c) your credentials
    d) the strength of peroxide being used   _____

17. A complete client record card should include:
    a) the client's signature
    b) hairstyle desired
    c) scalp condition
    d) amount of hair cut   _____

18. A release statement is used mainly to explain:
    a) your limited liability for haircolor mistakes
    b) if hair is in proper condition to receive color
    c) your malpractice insurance policy
    d) what the client may not sue for   _____

19. A predisposition test is performed to determine:
    a) haircolor results
    b) proper application method
    c) processing time
    d) allergy to aniline   _____

20. Red, yellow, and blue are considered:
    a) warm colors
    b) secondary colors
    c) primary colors
    d) cool colors   _____

21. The darkest primary color is:
    a) violet
    b) red
    c) blue
    d) yellow   _____

22. The equal combination of yellow and blue creates:
    a) orange
    b) green
    c) a tertiary color
    d) a warm color   _____

23. A complementary color combination is:
    a) red and orange
    b) red and yellow
    c) red and violet
    d) red and green   _____

24. If a client has unwanted orange tones, use a haircolor with a _____ base.
    a) violet
    b) blue
    c) green
    d) yellow   _____

25. Haircolors are divided into five classifications based on their:
    a) price
    b) staying power
    c) developer strength
    d) intensity
    _____

26. Temporary haircolor:
    a) makes a physical change
    b) requires a strand test
    c) penetrates the cortex
    d) lasts 4–6 shampoos
    _____

27. Semi-permanent color:
    a) requires a developer
    b) is only used with a pre-lightener
    c) will fade without a regrowth
    d) lasts 4–6 weeks
    _____

28. Semi-permanent color molecules are:
    a) larger than temporary
    b) only able to coat the cuticle
    c) smaller than permanent color
    d) smaller than temporary color
    _____

29. Semi-permanent color may not be used to:
    a) lighten the hair one level
    b) blend unpigmented hair
    c) tone pre-lightened hair
    d) deposit color
    _____

30. Polymer semi-permanent color may require:
    a) an oxidizer
    b) the use of heat
    c) pre-conditioning
    d) a double application
    _____

31. Non-ammonia alkali and a low volume developer are used with:
    a) polymer semi-permanent color
    b) oxidative deposit-only color
    c) traditional semi-permanent color
    d) non-oxidative permanent color
    _____

32. Henna is a form of:
    a) semi-permanent color
    b) metallic dye
    c) oxidative tint
    d) vegetable tint
    _____

33. Progressive haircolors and color restorers fall under the classification of:
    a) vegetable tints
    b) compound dyes
    c) metallic dyes
    d) oxidative tints
    _____

34. Para-dyes and penetrating tints fall into the category of:
    a) oxidative color
    b) semi-permanent color
    c) deposit-only color
    d) non-oxidative color _____

35. To create a certain degree of lift, tints contain:
    a) developer
    b) ammonia
    c) an oxidizer
    d) aniline _____

36. Oxidative tints work by:
    a) coating the cuticle
    b) coating the cortex
    c) swelling the hair shaft
    d) becoming trapped in
       the cuticle _____

37. The most commonly used oxidizer in haircoloring is:
    a) ammonia
    b) hydrogen peroxide
    c) oxygen
    d) aniline _____

38. Cream haircolor is generally applied with:
    a) bottle technique
    b) gloved hands
    c) foil
    d) brush-and-bowl _____

39. Dry peroxide is used to:
    a) boost peroxide strength
    b) dilute peroxide strength
    c) decrease processing time
    d) thicken liquid haircolor _____

40. A disadvantage of cream peroxide is it:
    a) may dry too quickly
    b) is hard to mix with color
    c) can become lumpy
    d) may dilute the color strength _____

41. A preliminary strand test should be performed:
    a) at the nape
    b) if the client requests it
    c) in the lower crown
    d) if the hair is to be cut _____

42. Once a temporary color rinse has been applied:
    a) rinse with warm water
    b) apply plastic cap
    c) apply conditioner
    d) style as desired _____

43. When selecting a semi-permanent color for hair that has no unpigmented hair, select a shade
   a) that matches the desired color
   b) two levels darker than the desired color
   c) one level darker than the desired color
   d) two levels lighter than the desired color _____

44. When formulating for semi-permanent haircolor, half of the formula is:
   a) the client's skin tone
   b) the natural hair color
   c) the client's eye color
   d) the last color used _____

45. As the volumes of oxygen are set free in hydrogen peroxide it becomes:
   a) water
   b) stronger
   c) ammonia
   d) hydrogen _____

46. Hydrogen peroxide should not come in contact with metal because:
   a) the metal will rust
   b) the peroxide will be too weak to work properly
   c) oxidation will not occur
   d) the peroxide strength will be increased _____

47. To lighten previously tinted hair,:
   a) select a lighter single-process tint
   b) apply powder bleach
   c) use a higher volume of peroxide
   d) use a color remover before tinting _____

48. A level 10 haircolor has less:
   a) lifting ability
   b) warmth
   c) ability to deposit base color
   d) need for ammonia _____

49. Hair at the scalp will process faster due to body heat and:
   a) more open cuticle layers
   b) incomplete keratinization
   c) larger cuticle scales
   d) incomplete melanin growth _____

50. Diluted color formula is applied to hair ends during a retouch procedure only if:
   a) it has been more than four weeks between retouches
   b) lightening the color
   c) required by the manufacturer
   d) the color is faded _____

51. During a hair lightening service, the hair becomes:
    a) finer
    b) more resistant
    c) coarser
    d) curlier
    _____

52. In a double-process lightener application, the lightener is followed by the application of:
    a) a toner
    b) dye remover
    c) a presoftener
    d) bleach
    _____

53. Oil bleach may be used to:
    a) lift four or more levels
    b) presoften resistant hair
    c) perform a tint back
    d) remove old haircolor
    _____

54. Cream lighteners may be mixed with dry crystals known as:
    a) accelerators
    b) dry ammonia
    c) oxidizers
    d) drabbers
    _____

55. The highest volume of peroxide used with lighteners is:
    a) 10
    b) 30
    c) 20
    d) 40
    _____

56. Increasing the number of dry crystal packets in a cream lightener formula will:
    a) weaken the product
    b) increase the strength of the lightener
    c) break the hair
    d) be determined by the length of the client's hair
    _____

57. Powder bleaches cannot be applied to:
    a) hair darker than a level 5
    b) gray hair
    c) hair darker than a level 3
    d) the scalp
    _____

58. Lighteners work by:
    a) removing melanin
    b) diffusing melanin
    c) lightening melanin
    d) toning melanin
    _____

59. Lightening may alter the hair's porosity, elasticity, and:
    a) texture
    b) future melanin production
    c) form
    d) length
    _____

60. There are _____ degrees of decolorizing.
    a) 4
    b) 10
    c) 7
    d) 2   _____

61. It is never safe to:
    a) process a lightener for
       60 minutes
    b) use any product with
       peroxide after a lightener
    c) remove a lightening mixture
       then reapply another
    d) bleach hair to white   _____

62. Lightener subsections should be:
    a) 1/8" inch
    b) 1/2" inch
    c) 1/4" inch
    d) 1" inch   _____

63. Lightener overlapping can cause breakage and:
    a) retard hair growth
    b) spot lightening
    c) lines of demarcation
    d) scalp irritation   _____

64. Before using a toner, the proper _____ must be achieved.
    a) level
    b) tone
    c) texture
    d) foundation   _____

65. It is common to use a _____ lightener when
    performing a cap highlighting technique.
    a) oil
    b) powder
    c) cream
    d) liquid   _____

66. Placing a lightener directly onto dry, styled hair is known as the:
    a) cap technique
    b) foil technique
    c) freehand technique
    d) freestyle technique   _____

67. To avoid affecting untreated hair during a highlighting treatment,
    use _____ when toning.
    a) high-lift tint
    b) nonoxidative toner
    c) filler
    d) a toner with
       20 volume peroxide   _____

68. To correct unwanted yellow tones in unpigmented hair, the
    colorist may apply:
    a) a blue rinse
    b) a neutral filler
    c) a lighter yellow tint
    d) a comparable level of violet _____

69. Presoftening is performed to open the cuticle and: 343
    a) open the cortex
    c) create missing gold tones
    b) eliminate gold tones
    d) soften melanin _____

70. To remove henna buildup, apply 70% alcohol for 5–7 344
    minutes, then:
    a) apply mineral oil
    c) rinse and shampoo
    b) apply desired tint
    d) rinse and apply cream bleach_____

71. The most effective way to guarantee future chemical services
    after the hair has been treated with metallic and coating dyes 346
    is to:
    a) use a dye solvent
    c) treat with 70% alcohol
    b) cut the tinted hair off
    d) apply ammonia water _____

72. Fillers are used to equalize porosity and: 348
    a) open the cuticle
    c) deposit a base color
    b) diffuse melanin
    d) remove color buildup _____

73. To achieve reds on darker natural levels, you may: 349
    a) prelighten
    c) presoften
    b) recommend hats
    d) use a high-lift red _____

74. Tint removal may be performed if: 350
    a) the color is too light
    c) the hair will not absorb toner
    b) the color is too dark
    d) bleach did not lift enough _____

75. After using a color remover:
    a) proceed with styling
    c) tint to desired color
    b) apply lightener
    d) perform foil highlighting _____

76. When performing a tint back,: 353
    a) a lightener should be used
    c) the hair should be
       presoftened
    b) the hair may need to be
       cut
    d) a filler may be used _____

77. The hair texture that may process slightly lighter when deposit-
    ing color is:
    a) fine
    c) gray
    b) coarse
    d) straight _____

78. Curlier hair may:
    a) reflect more light
    c) not lighten easily
    b) appear lighter
    d) require a stronger tone _____

79. The degree of darkness or lightness of a color is known as its:
    a) level
    c) tone
    b) intensity
    d) strength _____

80. The natural hair color "S" category indicates:
    a) dark hair
    c) light hair
    b) medium hair
    d) very light hair _____

81. The strongest intensity of pigmentation is found in the:
    a) "R" category
    c) "S" category
    b) "B" category
    d) "W" category _____

82. Unpigmented hair may be coarser and:
    a) more elastic
    c) straighter
    b) finer
    d) less elastic _____

83. During the consultation, it is best to select:
    a) the exact shade desired
    c) a color close to the natural color
    b) a general range of color
    d) directly from a paper chart _____

84. Swelling occurs in the hair shaft when using semi-permanent color due to the presence of:
    a) an alkali
    c) certified colors
    b) protinators
    d) hydrogen peroxide _____

85. Compound dyes are a combination of metallic dyes and:
    a) an oxidation tint
    c) polymers
    b) aniline
    d) vegetable tints _____

86. After an oxidation tint has been mixed and used, it:
    a) should be discarded
    c) is safe to use for 24 hours
    b) should be tightly sealed
    d) becomes a semi-permanent color _____

87. Permanent colors do not contain:
    a) a color base
    c) an aniline derivative
    b) hydrogen peroxide
    d) ammonia _____

88. When formulating permanent color for hair that is 10–30% unpigmented, your color choice should be:
    a) 2 parts desired level and 1 part lighter level
    c) equal parts desired and lighter level
    b) 1 level lighter
    d) level desired _____

89. The coating action of henna:
    a) may prevent penetration of other chemicals
    c) may increase penetration of other chemicals
    b) may leave a green cast
    d) can be tested with ammonia _____

90. When selecting a color filler:
    a) replace the hair's missing primary color
    c) replace the hair's missing secondary color
    b) reduce the additional primary color
    d) reduce the additional secondary color _____

91. The first step to properly camouflage excessive brassiness is:
    a) perform a patch test
    c) remove tint with dye remover
    b) identify actual color of brassiness
    d) use a violet based tint _____

92. A soap cap involves using shampoo with:
    a) oil bleach
    c) tint
    b) filler
    d) a color rinse _____

93. When a lightener is applied above the line of demarcation:
    a) a toner is required
    c) a soap cap is required
    b) breakage may occur
    d) the hair may not accept color _____

94. The underlying color that emerges during lightening is known as:
    a) pheomelanin
    c) undertone
    b) eumelanin
    d) intensity _____

95. If properly stored, peroxide maintains its strength for:
    a) 3 years
    c) 6 months
    b) 1 year
    d) 10 years _____

96. If hair is overlightened, the toner may make the hair appear:
   a) too light   c) white
   b) gray or ashy   d) too gold   _____

97. Color placed on damage hair may process:
   a) warmer   c) cooler
   b) lighter   d) slowly   _____

98. A highlighting shampoo is a combination of shampoo and:
   a) an aniline derivative tint   c) an oil bleach   340
   b) a semi-permanent tint   d) hydrogen peroxide   _____

99. An example of a double-process color application is:
   a) shampoo and apply   c) condition then apply toner
      temporary color
   b) spot lightening   d) presoften then tint _____

100. Polymer colors are classified as:
   a) temporary   c) semi-permanent
   b) deposit-only   d) oxidative tints   _____

Chemical Hair Relaxing and Soft-Curl Permanent

1. When using sodium hydroxide, protect the client's scalp with:
    a) gel
    b) stabilizer
    c) petroleum cream
    d) conditioner   _____

2. The action of a sodium hydroxide relaxer causes the hair to:
    a) soften and swell
    b) expand and harden
    c) harden and set
    d) shrink   _____

3. The chemical often required in addition to the chemical relaxer is:
    a) petroleum cream
    b) conditioner
    c) waving lotion
    d) stabilizer   _____

4. A product used to protect overporous or slightly damaged hair from being overprocessed on any part of the hair shaft is the:
    a) oxidizer
    b) activator
    c) conditioner/filler
    d) patch test   _____

5. To predetermine the results of a chemical relaxing treatment, it may be necessary to take a:
    a) patch test
    b) swatch test
    c) predisposition test
    d) strand test   _____

6. If the hair is damaged by hot-comb straightening, tinting, or lightening, the cosmetologist should:
    a) give the relaxer, then condition
    b) refuse to give the relaxer until conditioning treatments are given
    c) give the relaxer, then retint
    d) retint the hair, then give the relaxer   _____

7. A factor that affects the processing time of a chemical relaxer is:
   a) previous styling products used
   b) brand of relaxer used
   c) the client's age
   d) hair porosity

   _____

8. The scalp and skin are protected from possible burns when using a hair relaxer by applying:
   a) cotton
   b) a stabilizer
   c) an acid shampoo
   d) a base

   _____

9. After the hair has been processed with a sodium hydroxide relaxer and before the shampoo, the hair should be thoroughly:
   a) oiled
   b) rinsed
   c) dried
   d) conditioned

   _____

10. Before applying a thio relaxer, the hair may require:
    a) presoftening
    b) stabilizing
    c) a predisposition test
    d) a pre-shampoo

    _____

11. The relaxer cream is applied near the scalp last because processing is accelerated in this area by:
    a) your speed in application
    b) the sebaceous glands
    c) body heat
    d) perspiration

    _____

12. Combing tangles roughly from the hair after a chemical relaxing treatment may cause hair:
    a) reversion
    b) breakage
    c) discoloration
    d) knotting

    _____

13. The test that determines the hair's degree of elasticity is known as the _____ test.
    a) finger
    b) match
    c) pull
    d) strand

    _____

14. The best type of shampoo to use after the chemical relaxer is a/an:
    a) organic shampoo
    b) neutralizing shampoo
    c) antibacterial shampoo
    d) dry shampoo

    _____

15. After a chemical relaxing treatment, a hair conditioner is applied:
    a) before styling the hair   c) to the scalp only
    b) only if breakage is present   d) to the ends only   _____

16. When analyzing hair condition, it is necessary to evaluate the hair's porosity, texture, and:
    a) style   c) cut
    b) color   d) elasticity   _____

17. The two commonly used methods of chemical hair relaxing are the thio method and the _____ method.
    a) thermal   c) hard press
    b) sodium hydroxide   d) ammonium thioglycolate   _____

18. A hair relaxing treatment should be avoided when an examination shows the presence of:
    a) pityriasis   c) prior styling products
    b) scalp abrasions   d) excessive oils   _____

19. *Hair porosity* refers to the ability of the hair to:
    a) accept stabilizer   c) stretch and return
    b) dry quickly   d) absorb moisture   _____

20. *Hair elasticity* refers to the ability of the hair to:
    a) grow without shedding   c) absorb moisture
    b) stretch and return   d) regrow after breakage   _____

21. *Hair texture* refers to the hair's:
    a) fullness or flatness   c) coarseness or fineness
    b) amount per square inch   d) ability to stretch and return _____

22. The three general methods for applying chemical hair relaxer are the comb method, the brush method, and:
    a) the glove method   c) the foil method
    b) the cap method   d) the finger method   _____

23. To check relaxer processing, press a strand to the scalp, if the hair "beads" from the scalp,:
    a) rinse immediately   c) add neutralizer
    b) continue to process   d) mist with water bottle   _____

24. A blow-out style is a combination of hairstyling and:
    a) chemical overprocessing
    b) clipper cutting
    c) chemical straightening
    d) elevated cutting
    _____

25. An implement needed to perform a chemical blow-out is a:
    a) blow dryer
    b) teasing comb
    c) thermal iron
    d) heat lamp
    _____

26. When performing a chemical blow-out, the important consideration is that the hair must *not* be:
    a) air waved
    b) overrelaxed
    c) underrelaxed
    d) lifted
    _____

27. The natural oils removed by the relaxer are replaced by:
    a) shampooing
    b) stabilizing
    c) rinsing
    d) conditioning
    _____

28. Soft-curl permanent waving is a method of:
    a) permanent waving straight hair
    b) permanent waving overly curly hair
    c) permanently relaxing the hair
    d) relaxing permanently waved hair
    _____

29. A soft-curl permanent should *not* be given to hair that is:
    a) relaxed with sodium hydroxide
    b) not ethnic hair
    c) relaxed with ammonium thioglycolate
    d) overly curly
    _____

30. Thio gel or cream, used in giving a soft-curl perm, is applied to the hair in order to:
    a) increase scalp flexibility
    b) harden the hair before processing
    c) soften the hair for wrapping
    d) harden the hair for wrapping
    _____

31. In order to arrange the curl pattern, the rods selected for a soft-curl permanent should be:
    a) at least 2 times larger than the natural curl
    b) 1 size smaller than the natural curl
    c) equal to the natural curl
    d) at least 2 times larger than the desired curl
    _____

32. In order to achieve good curl formation, the hair should circle the rod at least:
    a) 2 1/2 times
    b) 4 times
    c) 1 1/2 times
    d) 1 time
    _____

33. When giving a soft-curl perm, apply thio until all hair on rods is thoroughly saturated, then:
    a) mist with water
    b) rinse excess thio
    c) replace saturated cotton
    d) drape the client
    _____

34. After properly neutralizing a soft-curl perm, it is important to:
    a) remove rods carefully
    b) rinse with hot water
    c) leave hair on rods until dry
    d) apply base
    _____

35. After a soft-curl perm, a/an_____ may be used to maintain the sheen of the hair.
    a) neutralizer
    b) activator
    c) developer
    d) water rinse
    _____

Thermal Hair Straightening

1. Hair pressing generally lasts:
   a) overnight
   b) until shampooed
   c) one week
   d) from haircut to haircut _____

2. Types of hair pressing are the soft press, hard press, and:
   a) croquignole press
   b) light press
   c) figure 8 press
   d) medium press _____

3. The temperature of the pressing comb should be adjusted to the hair's:
   a) cleanliness
   b) style
   c) texture
   d) length _____

4. The best time to give a hair press is:
   a) before a shampoo
   b) after a shampoo
   c) before the hair is oiled
   d) after a styling _____

5. The least difficult type of hair to press is:
   a) wiry, curly hair
   b) resistant, curly hair
   c) virgin hair
   d) medium curly hair _____

6. When pressing gray hair, use light pressure and:
   a) moderate heat
   b) more pressing oil
   c) intense heat
   d) a larger pressing comb _____

7. Hair that appears lifeless and limp is usually lacking in:
   a) elasticity
   b) texture
   c) porosity
   d) density _____

8. The type of hair that requires the least heat and pressure is:
   a) coarse
   b) fine
   c) short
   d) curly _____

9. Applying a heated comb twice on each side of the hair is known as a:
   a) hard press
   b) soft press
   c) regular press
   d) comb press _____

10. Hair pressing:
    a) permanently waves hair
    b) temporarily curls straight hair
    c) temporarily straightens hair
    d) gives wide waves to curly hair _____

11. A good hair pressing treatment:
    a) improves hair texture
    b) is not harmful to hair
    c) improves hair condition
    d) lasts 4–6 weeks _____

12. A press is given with:
    a) marcel irons
    b) protective cream
    c) a scalp massage
    d) a pressing comb _____

13. If the pressing comb is not hot enough, the hair will:
    a) require more pressure
    b) not straighten
    c) require more pressing oil
    d) need a double press _____

14. Burnt hair strands:
    a) only occur in a hard press
    b) seal in oil
    c) cannot be conditioned
    d) help hold certain styles _____

15. In pressing coarse hair, more heat is required because it:
    a) contains a medulla
    b) has the greatest diameter
    c) has an enlarged cuticle
    d) is never gray _____

16. When given a hair press, coarse, overly curly hair can tolerate:
    a) less heat than fine hair
    b) less pressure than medium hair
    c) less pressing oil
    d) more heat than fine hair _____

17. To avoid breakage when pressing fine hair, the following is required:
    a) more heat and pressure
    b) less heat and pressure
    c) more protective cream
    d) no pressing oil _____

18. The use of excess heat on gray, tinted, or lightened hair may:
    a) alter future hair growth
    b) make the hair wiry
    c) discolor the hair
    d) ruin the pressing comb _____

19. Failure to correct dry and brittle hair before thermal straightening may result in:
    a) hair breakage
    b) a weaker result
    c) more retouch treatments
    d) overcurling _____

20. To avoid smoke or burning while pressing hair, use:
    a) more heat
    b) preheated pressing oil
    c) less pressing oil
    d) more pressing oil _____

21. A hard press in which a hot curling iron is passed through the hair first is called:
    a) a chemical press
    b) a double press
    c) a thermal press
    d) a rod press _____

22. Hair pressing treatments between shampoos are called:
    a) touch-ups
    b) re-do's
    c) re-presses
    d) soft presses _____

23. When pressing lightened or tinted hair, use light pressure and:
    a) more heat
    b) moderate heat
    c) less pressing oil
    d) a protective base _____

24. Wiry, overly curly hair has qualities that make it:
    a) easiest to press
    b) require less pressing oil
    c) difficult to press
    d) necessary to relax before a pressing treatment _____

25. Before performing a hair press, the hair should be sectioned in:
    a) 9 sections
    b) 4 sections
    c) 5 sections
    d) 3 sections _____

26. A scalp may be classified as normal, flexible, or:
    a) brittle   c) porous
    b) thin   d) tight   _____

27. Applying the thermal pressing comb once on each side of the
    hair is required for a:
    a) soft press   c) croquignole press
    b) double press   d) hard press   _____

28. Pressing combs should be constructed of good-quality steel or:
    a) zinc   c) plastic
    b) hard rubber   d) brass   _____

29. The actual pressing or straightening of the hair is accomplished
    with the comb's:
    a) teeth   c) back rod
    b) handle   d) tail   _____

30. Hair and scalp may be reconditioned with special hair products,
    hair brushing, and:
    a) intense rinsing   c) a lemon rinse
    b) a dry shampoo   d) a scalp massage   _____

31. The metal portion of a pressing comb may be immersed in a
    solution of _____ for 1 hour to give it a smooth
    and shiny appearance.
    a) ammonia   c) sodium hypochlorite
    b) hot baking soda   d) alcohol and shampoo   _____

32. When giving a pressing treatment, the cosmetologist should
    avoid:
    a) excessive heat and pressure   c) the hair ends
    b) thoroughly drying the hair   d) sectioning the hair   _____

33. Too frequent hair pressing treatments can cause:
    a) excessive oiliness of hair   c) progressive hair breakage
    b) hirsuties   d) hypertrichosis   _____

34. Carbon may be removed from the pressing comb by rubbing
    with:
    a) a wet towel   c) disinfectant
    b) an emery board   d) pressing oil   _____

The Artistry of Artificial Hair

1. Modacrylic is a term used to describe wigs made from:
   a) animal hair
   b) human hair
   c) synthetic fibers
   d) a blend of animal and human hair

   _____

2. Human hair wigs may be colored with a color rinse that:
   a) lasts permanently
   b) does not deposit color
   c) lightens the color
   d) lasts from cleaning to cleaning

   _____

3. Human hair wigs can be distinguished from synthetic hair wigs by a simple:
   a) pull test
   b) match test
   c) predisposition test
   d) strand test

   _____

4. Human hair wigs may be properly cleaned with:
   a) a liquid cleanser
   b) any shampoo
   c) an alkaline soap
   d) dry shampoo only

   _____

5. If human hair wigs are worn frequently, they should be cleaned every:
   a) 2–4 weeks
   b) 8–10 weeks
   c) 2–3 months
   d) 4–6 months

   _____

6. Dryness or brittleness of wigs is prevented by:
   a) storing on a cork block
   b) rarely brushing
   c) conditioning
   d) dry shampooing

   _____

7. Wig styles are kept close to the head by using:
   a) smaller rollers
   b) pin curls
   c) larger rollers
   d) barrel curls

   _____

8. A long weft of hair mounted with a loop at the end is known as a:
   a) demi-wig
   b) fall
   c) switch
   d) chignon
   _____

9. A hairpiece with a flat base that blends with the client's own hair is a:
   a) cascade
   b) fall
   c) bandeau
   d) wiglet
   _____

10. Each time a human hair wig is cleaned, it should be:
   a) resized
   b) reconditioned
   c) reknotted
   d) restretched
   _____

11. To shorten a wig from front to nape, it is advisable to use:
   a) horizontal tucks
   b) stronger elastic
   c) vertical tucks
   d) a smaller block and hot water to shrink the base
   _____

12. To remove width at the back of the wig from ear to ear, use:
   a) horizontal tucks
   b) stronger elastic
   c) a smaller block and hot water to shrink the base
   d) vertical tucks
   _____

13. The type of head block that is suitable for all wig services is a:
   a) metal block
   b) porcelain block
   c) canvas block
   d) Styrofoam block
   _____

14. Hand-tied wigs should be cleaned:
   a) in a non-metal bowl
   b) on a block
   c) less frequently
   d) every 3 months
   _____

15. When cutting a human hair wig, special care must be taken to:
   a) keep the hair dry
   b) never use a razor
   c) keep the cap dry
   d) decrease bulk
   _____

Manicuring and Pedicuring

1. Emery boards are used to:
   a) thin the free edge
   b) remove dirt from under the nail
   c) shape the free edge
   d) push back the cuticle

   C

2. Nail shapes should conform to the client's:
   a) hand size
   b) fingertips
   c) nail bed
   d) free edge

   B

3. If blood is drawn during a procedure, the implement should be:
   a) discarded
   b) wiped off with cotton
   c) cleaned and disinfected
   d) rinsed with water

   C

4. Brittle nails and dry cuticles are treated with a/an:
   a) oil manicure
   b) hand massage
   c) cuticle pusher
   d) extended soaking time

   A

5. If a client is accidentally cut during a manicure, apply:
   a) styptic pencil
   b) powdered alum
   c) pressure
   d) alcohol

   B

6. A nail hardener is applied:
   a) after the base coat
   b) before the base coat
   c) after the nail polish
   d) after the top coat

   B

7. A manicure that is not given in the manicuring area, and often is given while the client is receiving another service, is called a:
   a) booth manicure
   b) hot oil manicure
   c) plain manicure
   d) mobile manicure

   A

8. Fresh disinfectant solution for implements should be prepared:
   a) weekly
   b) daily
   c) every 2 days
   d) 3 times a day

    B

9. Polish should be removed with:
   a) a firm movement from the base of the nail to the tip
   b) a twisting motion
   c) a firm movement from the tip of the nail to the base
   d) a circular motion –

   A

10. When shaping the fingernail, the nail is filed from:
    a) corner to center
    b) left to right
    c) center to corner
    d) corner to corner

    A

11. When trimming the cuticle, be sure to remove it:
    a) in small sections
    b) on one side at a time
    c) as a single segment
    d) at the base only

    C

12. All traces of oil must be removed after an oil manicure before:
    a) filing
    b) applying the base coat
    c) massage
    d) applying the top coat

    B

13. The correct way to apply nail polish from base to free edge is to:
    a) work from the sides to the center
    b) use short strokes
    c) allow the polish to form a ball on the brush before spreading
    d) apply it quickly and lightly

    D

14. A hand massage may be given before:
    a) polish
    b) soaking fingers
    c) filing
    d) pushing cuticles

    A

15. Once polish has been applied, wipe away excess with:
    a) your thumbnail
    b) a cuticle pusher
    c) a cotton-tipped orangewood stick
    d) a cotton pledget

    C

16. Apply nail polish:
    a) over the top coat
    b) over the base coat
    c) over the sealer
    d) before the base coat

     B

17. The ideal nail shape is:
    a) tapered
    b) rectangular
    c) oval
    d) round

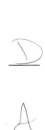
c

18. Stains on fingernails may be removed with nail bleach or:
    a) an oil manicure
    b) pumice powder
    c) acetone
    d) peroxide

D

19. Wavy ridges may be improved by buffing the nail with:
    a) pumice powder
    b) a metal file
    c) oil
    d) a filing block

A

20. To mend torn, broken, or split nails, and to fortify weak or fragile nails, the following service is recommended:
    a) oil manicure
    b) nail filing
    c) nail wrapping
    d) cuticle pushing

    _____

21. A nail buffer may not be used:
    a) on the natural nail
    b) with dry polish
    c) where not permitted by law
    d) with pumice powder

    _____

22. To keep the client's hands well groomed and smooth, each manicure should include:
    a) hot oil
    b) cuticle removal
    c) pumice powder
    d) a hand massage

    _____

23. For clients with ridged and brittle nails or dry cuticles, recommend a/an:
    a) oil manicure
    b) longer soaking time
    c) square nail shape
    d) nail wrapping

    _____

24. Brushes used for acrylic overlay are cleaned by dipping into:
    a) alcohol
    b) soapy water
    c) a weak quat
    d) polish remover

    _____

25. What material should never be used on plastic artificial nails?
    a) cuticle oil
    b) nail polish dryer
    c) acetone polish remover
    d) hand lotion

    _____

26. Nail wraps using silk allow:
    a) the most strength
    b) easy application
    c) easy removal
    d) a smooth, even appearance _____

27. The strongest material used for nail wrapping is:
    a) mending tissue
    b) acrylic
    c) silk
    d) linen _____

28. A stick of nail bleach is wiped:
    a) over the nail bed
    b) on top of the free edge
    c) under the free edge
    d) around the cuticle _____

29. When applying acrylic, the first ball should be placed:
    a) at the free edge
    b) at the base of the nail
    c) in the middle of the nail
    d) at one side of the nail _____

30. Nail antiseptic is applied to nails receiving sculptured nail fill-ins immediately before:
    a) filing
    b) cleaning nails
    c) primer
    d) polish _____

31. To help prevent contamination in an acrylic nail service, do not touch the nail:
    a) while tacky with base coat
    b) with bare hands
    c) after primer is applied
    d) after dust and filings are removed _____

32. Removal of any artificial nail product can cause damage to the natural nail if the manicurist:
    a) uses oily polish remover
    b) pulls or twists the product
    c) uses acetone polish remover
    d) uses an orangewood stick _____

33. Pumice powder is likely to be an ingredient found in a:
    a) cuticle cream
    b) nail abrasive
    c) hand cream
    d) dry nail polish _____

34. A simple method to add length rather than strength may be accomplished by:
    a) nail wrapping
    b) liquid nail treatments
    c) an acrylic overlay
    d) nail tipping _____

35. A buffer block is used during a sculptured nail fill or repair to:
    a) buff acrylic and blend it into the new growth area
    b) thin out the free edge
    c) thin the nail plate
    d) reshape the free edge _____

36. The trapping of dirt and _____ between artificial nail products and the natural nail may lead to fungus.
    a) nail polish
    b) primer
    c) moisture
    d) natural nail oils _____

37. A top coat or sealer makes the nail polish:
    a) adhere to the nail surface
    b) more resistant to chipping
    c) appear thicker
    d) dry quickly _____

38. The finger bowl should be filled with
    a) cuticle cream
    b) antibacterial soap
    c) disinfectant
    d) dry nail polish _____

39. Most artificial nail adhesives are:
    a) a gel
    b) not to be used with plastic
    c) flammable
    d) a cause of nail fungus _____

40. If a client has athlete's foot, recommend:
    a) a medicated shoe insert
    b) a pedicure
    c) changing socks more frequently
    d) a physician's examination _____

41. To avoid ingrown nails:
    a) be sure nails are rounded
    b) do not file into the corners
    c) be sure nails have a 1/4" free edge
    d) use the fine side of the emery board _____

42. If offering a leg massage with a pedicure, do not massage:
    a) the muscular tissue on the side of the shinbone
    b) above the ankle
    c) the shinbone
    d) below the knee _____

43. A physician who specializes in foot care is known as a/an:
    a) dermatologist
    b) podiatrist
    c) orthopedic physician
    d) opthomologist _____

44. When applying press-on artificial nails, do not apply adhesive:
    a) on the edges of the natural nail
    b) until the nail is applied
    c) to the inside of the artificial nail
    d) on the center of the nail   _____

45. When performing a pedicure:
    a) do not massage toes
    b) the cuticle is not cut
    c) do not use astringent
    d) do not apply base coat   _____

The Nail and Its Disorders

1. A healthy nail is smooth, curved, and without hollows or:
   - a) wavy ridges
   - b) flexibility
   - c) firmness
   - d) curves

   _____

2. A healthy nail appears:
   - a) purplish
   - b) pinkish
   - c) yellowish
   - d) bluish

   _____

3. The function of the nail is to:
   - a) adorn the fingertips
   - b) protect the matrix
   - c) give strength to the fingers
   - d) protect the fingertips

   _____

4. The nail is composed of keratin, which is:
   - a) a polypeptide bond
   - b) hard tissue
   - c) a protein
   - d) hardened epithelial cells

   _____

5. In an adult, nails grow at an average of:
   - a) 1/8" per month
   - b) 1/8" per week
   - c) 1/2" per month
   - d) 1/4" per week

   _____

6. Nails tend to grow faster:
   - a) in the winter
   - b) on elderly people
   - c) on children
   - d) in the spring

   _____

7. The nail plate is also known as the:
   - a) mantle
   - b) nail bed
   - c) free edge
   - d) nail body

   _____

8. The nail root is lodged in a growing tissue known as the:
   a) nail body
   b) mantle
   c) nail plate
   d) matrix
   _____

9. _____ is a nail condition that may receive a manicure.
   a) Onychosis
   b) Onychophagy
   c) Onychia
   d) Paronychia
   _____

10. The part of the nail that extends over the fingertip is the:
    a) free edge
    b) matrix
    c) hyponychium
    d) lunula
    _____

11. Cells that generate and harden the nail are found in the:
    a) nail body
    b) nail plate
    c) nail bed
    d) matrix
    _____

12. The light color of the lunula is caused by the reflection of light where:
    a) the free edge and nail bed meet
    b) the matrix and the connective tissue of the nail bed join
    c) the matrix and the cuticle join
    d) the nail bed and the nail walls join
    _____

13. The nail matrix:
    a) does not affect nail strength
    b) is constantly reproducing
    c) contains no nerves
    d) is responsible for nail color   _____

14. The lunula's shape is:
    a) triangular
    b) oval
    c) half-moon
    d) round
    _____

15. The technical name for the nail is:
    a) onychosis
    b) onyx
    c) onychauxis
    d) onychia
    _____

16. The cuticle overlapping the lunula is the:
    a) hyponychium
    b) eponychium
    c) perionychium
    d) nail wall
    _____

17. Replacement of an entire nail takes approximately:
    a) 4 weeks
    c) 2 months
    b) 6 weeks
    d) 4 months _____

18. The deep fold of skin in which the nail root is embedded is the:
    a) matrix
    c) mantle
    b) nail wall
    d) nail groove _____

19. If the matrix is destroyed, the nail will:
    a) become harder
    c) grow faster
    b) not grow back
    d) grow slower _____

20. The overlapping part of the skin around the nail is commonly called the nail:
    a) hyponychium
    c) mantle
    b) leuconychia
    d) cuticle _____

21. The portion of the skin under the free edge is called the:
    a) hyponychium
    c) perionychium
    b) eponychium
    d) cuticle _____

22. The extension of the cuticle skin at the base of the nail is known as the:
    a) hyponychium
    c) perionychium
    b) eponychium
    d) nail bed _____

23. The nail walls are small folds of skin overlapping the sides of the:
    a) mantle
    c) bed
    b) free edge
    d) nail body _____

24. The nail grooves are the furrowed tracks at the:
    a) sides of the nail
    c) root of the nail
    b) base of the nail
    d) mantle of the nail _____

25. White spots on the nails are known as:
    a) onychauxis
    c) leuconychia
    b) onychatrophia
    d) hangnails _____

26. When the cuticle splits around the nail, it is known as:
    a) onychorrhexis
    c) onychophagy
    b) hangnails
    d) pterygium _____

27. Blue nails are usually a sign of:
    a) wrist trouble
    b) a stomach ailment
    c) poor blood circulation
    d) a lung disorder _____

28. Wavy ridges on the nails are caused by:
    a) careless filing of the nails
    b) dryness of the cuticle
    c) uneven growth of the nails
    d) biting the nails _____

29. The common name for tinea is:
    a) ringworm
    b) ingrown nails
    c) felon
    d) hangnail _____

30. Hangnails may be caused by dryness of the:
    a) lunula
    b) matrix
    c) medulla
    d) cuticle _____

31. Splitting of the nails may be caused by:
    a) nail polish
    b) careless filing
    c) hangnails
    d) omytosis _____

32. An infectious and inflammatory condition of the tissues surrounding the nail is known as:
    a) onychatrophia
    b) paronychia
    c) onychia
    d) onychoptosis _____

33. Hangnails are treated by softening the cuticle with:
    a) hot oil
    b) primer
    c) a hot water fingerbath
    d) acetone _____

34. Furrows in the nails may be caused by:
    a) an allergy
    b) dermatitis
    c) illness
    d) nail polish _____

35. The forward and adhering growth of the cuticle at the base of the nail is called:
    a) atrophy
    b) pterygium
    c) paronychia
    d) onychosis _____

36. An infected finger should be treated by a/an:
    a) manicurist
    b) instructor
    c) physician
    d) cosmetologist _____

37. The general term for a vegetable parasite is:
    a) fungi   c) onychauxis
    b) flagella   d) onychosis   _____

38. The fungus infection caused when moisture is trapped between
    the unsanitized natural nail and artificial nail products is called:
    a) scabies   c) nail mold
    b) onyx   d) pterygium   _____

39. Advanced nail mold causes the nail to turn black and:
    a) harden   c) crumble
    b) smell bad   d) split   _____

40. Onychia is an inflammation with pus formation affecting the:
    a) nail body   c) free edge
    b) nail matrix   d) cuticle sides of the nail   _____

41. The technical term indicating any nail disease is:
    a) onychauxis   c) onychosis
    b) onyx   d) onychophagy   _____

42. If not properly cared for, hangnails may:
    a) cause corrugations   c) become infected
    b) cause onychauxis   d) become tinea   _____

43. Furrows may be caused by injury to the cells near the:
    a) free edge   c) walls
    b) matrix   d) grooves   _____

44. Eggshell nails are usually found on persons with a chronic:
    a) digestive disturbance   c) circulatory disturbance
    b) nervous disturbance   d) muscular disturbance   _____

45. An abnormal overgrowth of the nail is known as:
    a) atrophy   c) onychophagy
    b) hypertrophy   d) onychorrhexis   _____

46. The medical term for brittle nails is:
    a) onychorrhexis   c) hypertrophy
    b) onychophagy   d) atrophy   _____

47. The medical term for bitten nails is:
    a) leuconychia   c) onychauxis
    b) onychia   d) onychophagy   _____

48. Onychocryptosis is commonly called:
    a) felon   c) ingrown nails
    b) bitten nails   d) ringworm   _____

49. An overgrowth in the thickness of a nail is known as:
    a) onychatropia   c) onychophagy
    b) onychia   d) onychauxis   _____

50. The only service you may be allowed to perform for a client with
    nail fungus or mold is to:
    a) apply polish   c) buff to a shine
    b) remove any artificial nails   d) refill the new growth   _____

Theory of Massage

1. Effluerage, or stroking, is a massage movement applied in a:
   a) heavy tapping manner
   b) deep rolling manner with pressure
   c) light pinching manner
   d) light, slow, and rhythmic manner without firm pressure _____

2. Massage should not be given to clients with high blood pressure or a heart condition because it:
   a) requires them to lie flat
   b) increases muscular strength
   c) may become irritating
   d) increases circulation _____

3. Petrissage is what type of massage movement?
   a) kneading
   b) percussion
   c) tapotement
   d) friction _____

4. One area the cosmetologist is not licensed to massage is the:
   a) leg below the knee
   b) upper chest
   c) leg above the knee
   d) below the neck _____

5. Friction in massage requires the use of:
   a) vibratory movements
   b) slapping movements
   c) deep rubbing movements
   d) light stroking movements _____

6. When performing a stroking movement, the fingers:
   a) gently tap the skin
   b) are not used
   c) remain rigid
   d) conform to the shape of the area being massaged _____

7. To master massage techniques, you must have knowledge of anatomy and:
   a) psychology
   b) histology
   c) physiology
   d) chemistry
   _____

8. The fixed attachment of one end of a muscle to a bone or tissue is known as the _____ of a muscle.
   a) joint
   b) origin
   c) point
   d) insertion
   _____

9. Firm kneading massage movements usually produce:
   a) deep stimulation
   b) cooling sensations
   c) soothing sensations
   d) muscle contractions
   _____

10. Tapotement is a _____ massage movement.
    a) vibratory
    b) pinching
    c) friction
    d) tapping
    _____

11. Massage should not be given when:
    a) sunburn is present
    b) fillings are present
    c) abrasions are present
    d) tension is present
    _____

12. Chucking is an example of:
    a) kneading
    b) friction
    c) fulling
    d) petrissage
    _____

13. Manipulating proper motor points will:
    a) relax the client
    b) give the skin a glow
    c) provide the deepest stimulation
    d) warm the muscle for massage
    _____

14. Normal skin can be maintained by _____ massage.
    a) daily
    b) weekly
    c) monthly
    d) annual
    _____

15. Fulling is performed mainly on the:
    a) chin
    b) legs
    c) neck
    d) arms
    _____

16. Joint movements are restricted to the arms, hands, and:
    a) shoulders
    c) neck
    b) feet
    d) legs
    _____

17. The proper position of the fingers for effleurage is:
    a) flat
    c) slightly bent for pinching
    b) each finger must touch
    d) curved
    _____

18. The most invigorating massage movement is:
    a) kneading
    c) friction
    b) tapotement
    d) vibration
    _____

19. The gentlest massage movement is:
    a) petrissage
    c) fulling
    b) tapotement
    d) effleurage
    _____

20. Body contours or fatty tissues may be reduced over a period of time by using:
    a) firm kneading
    c) effleurage
    b) joint movements
    d) therapeutic lamps
    _____

Facials

1. The first cream or lotion to be used in a plain facial is:
   - a) an astringent lotion
   - b) massage cream
   - c) cleansing cream
   - d) moisturizing lotion _____

2. When a facial is given, eye pads should be applied before using:
   - a) infrared rays
   - b) astringent lotion
   - c) a facial steamer
   - d) a depilatory _____

3. When draping for a facial, a towel must be placed:
   - a) on the back of the facial chair
   - b) around the client's neck
   - c) around the client's feet
   - d) over the client's shoulders _____

4. Following the removal of blackheads, apply _____ to the skin.
   - a) a mud mask
   - b) massage cream
   - c) astringent
   - d) cool towels _____

5. No face powder or cheek color is applied after giving a/an:
   - a) steam treatment
   - b) extraction
   - c) hot wax treatment
   - d) acne treatment _____

6. The two basic types of facials are preservative and:
   - a) cleansing
   - b) moisturizing
   - c) corrective
   - d) acne _____

7. After the massage cream has been removed, the face should be sponged with a/an:
   - a) warm towel or cotton pledget
   - b) toner
   - c) cool water rinse
   - d) astringent lotion _____

8. If it is necessary to cleanse pimples that have come to a head and are open, the cosmetologist should use:
   a) a facial steamer
   b) gloves
   c) a cotton mask
   d) a sponge _____

9. Fine-textured skin may not allow:
   a) moisture to remain on the skin surface
   b) sebum to pass through to the skin surface
   c) moisture to penetrate the skin surface
   d) the formation of milia _____

10. Acne is a disorder of the sebaceous glands; therefore, it requires:
    a) alcohol treatments
    b) medicated facials
    c) medical attention
    d) a mask or pack with the facial _____

11. When skillfully applied, massage benefits the skin by:
    a) removing debris
    b) forcing cream into the skin
    c) warming the temperature of the body
    d) stimulation _____

12. For dry skin, avoid using lotions that contain a large percentage of:
    a) lanolin
    b) hormones
    c) alcohol
    d) oil _____

13. When receiving a facial, an important part for the client is:
    a) the angle of the chair
    b) relaxation
    c) conversation
    d) refreshments available _____

14. Overactive sebaceous glands produce too much:
    a) oil
    b) perspiration
    c) moisture
    d) pH _____

15. The direction of pressure in facial massage movements should be from the muscle:
    a) origin to insertion
    b) insertion to origin
    c) posterior to inferior
    d) superior to inferior _____

16. All items needed for a facial should be arranged:
    a) in size order
    b) before each client arrives
    c) according to price
    d) in the morning _____

17. Studies show that acne may be due to:
    a) chocolate
    b) lack of skin treatments
    c) fast foods
    d) hereditary factors   _____

18. Blackheads are caused by:
    a) dirt trapped in open pores
    b) heredity
    c) a hardened mass of sebum
    d) dietary factors   _____

19. Milia is a common skin disorder that often occurs in skin texture that is:
    a) coarse
    b) oily
    c) fine
    d) soft   _____

20. A yogurt or buttermilk mask has a _____ action.
    a) soothing
    b) mildly astringent
    c) toning
    d) hydrating   _____

21. The purpose of gauze in a facial is to:
    a) remove packs easily
    b) prevent mask from touching the skin
    c) hold mask ingredients together
    d) comply with sanitation laws _____

22. An egg facial mask will cleanse the pores and:
    a) lubricate the skin
    b) remove wrinkles
    c) soothe the skin
    d) tighten the skin   _____

23. A household ingredient that may be used for a hydrating effect in a mask is:
    a) strawberries
    b) egg whites
    c) cucumbers
    d) honey   _____

24. A banana mask leaves the skin:
    a) with an oily residue
    b) feeling refreshed
    c) soft and smooth
    d) slightly dry   _____

25. A client may not be happy with a facial service if:
    a) they do not hear soft music
    b) they are told about future promotions
    c) they see too many products
    d) the cosmetologist runs out of products _____

Facial Makeup

1. Proper draping for makeup should include:
   a) a terrycloth robe
   b) a cotton smock
   c) a sheet or blanket
   d) a headband or turban _____

2. The most important makeup is probably:
   a) mascara
   b) foundation
   c) translucent powder
   d) rouge _____

3. Face powder should be:
   a) cake style
   b) blendable with the color tone of the skin
   c) shiny when applied
   d) eliminated when using foundation _____

4. Cheek color (rouge) that blends well and is suitable for all skin types is:
   a) liquid
   b) dry
   c) cream
   d) powder _____

5. In corrective makeup, a lighter shade is used to:
   a) minimize a facial area
   b) widen or lengthen an area
   c) conceal blemishes
   d) emphasize a facial area _____

6. An astringent lotion is applied after tweezing eyebrows in order to:
   a) relax the skin
   b) contract the skin
   c) expand the skin
   d) stimulate the skin _____

7. The color of foundation is tested by blending on a patron's:
   a) jawline
   b) eyelid
   c) forehead
   d) wrist _____

8. Lipstick should be applied with a lip brush beginning:
   a) in the middle of the lower lip
   b) at the inner peak of the upper lip
   c) at the corner of the lower lip
   d) at the corner of the upper lip
   _____

9. The primary objective of corrective makeup is to create the optical illusion of a/an:
   a) oval face
   b) diamond-shaped face
   c) round face
   d) heart-shaped face
   _____

10. Translucent face powder is:
    a) darker than foundation
    b) colorless
    c) lighter than foundation
    d) the same color as foundation
    _____

11. Before applying foundation makeup,:
    a) the skin should be damp
    b) a face powder is applied
    c) the skin should be cleansed
    d) lipstick is selected
    _____

12. Eyeliner is used to make the:
    a) lash color match the brow color
    b) lashes look longer
    c) natural color of the iris appear darker
    d) eyes appear larger
    _____

13. The last cosmetic to be applied is usually:
    a) mascara
    b) face powder
    c) lipstick
    d) cheek color
    _____

14. Eyebrows are properly tweezed:
    a) in an upward movement
    b) in the direction of their natural growth
    c) after foundation is applied
    d) before every makeup application
    _____

15. Applying cotton saturated with hot water on the eyebrows before tweezing:
    a) eliminates redness
    b) softens and relaxes eyebrow tissue
    c) tightens the tissues
    d) contracts the skin
    _____

16. In corrective makeup, a darker shade is used to:
    a) emphasize a facial area
    b) minimize a facial area
    c) attract the eye
    d) broaden a facial area
    _____

17. When two shades of foundation are used, they must be blended to prevent:
    a) too much contrast
    b) an allergic reaction
    c) a line of demarcation
    d) the use of face powder   _____

18. To minimize wide-set eyes and make them appear closer, it is best to:
    a) shorten the outside eyebrow line on both sides
    b) extend the eyebrow line to inside the corner of the eye
    c) make the eyebrow line straight
    d) arch the ends of the eyebrow   _____

19. When choosing foundation color for light skin, select a shade _____ than the natural color.
    a) darker
    b) lighter
    c) beiger
    d) rosier   _____

20. Eye tabbing involves:
    a) applying strip eyelashes
    b) applying individual lashes
    c) tinting eyelashes
    d) removing artificial lashes   _____

21. Semi-permanent individual eyelashes are made of:
    a) human hair
    b) animal hair
    c) inorganic fibers
    d) synthetic fibers   _____

22. Semi-permanent individual eyelashes last for a period of:
    a) 6–8 weeks
    b) 3–6 months
    c) 2–3 weeks
    d) 7–14 days   _____

23. The individual lashes will not stay on as long on the lower lids because of:
    a) natural oils
    b) perspiration
    c) possible moisture from tears
    d) their shorter length   _____

24. A client with a heart-shaped face can be identified by:
    a) a narrow forehead
    b) a wide jawline
    c) a narrow jawline
    d) a high forehead   _____

The Skin and Its Disorders

1. The skin's feel and appearance is known as its:
   a) elasticity
   b) porosity
   c) texture
   d) density _____

2. Healthy skin is:
   a) free from nonpathogenic
      bacteria
   b) free of sebum
   c) slightly acid
   d) alkaline and firm _____

3. An indication of a good complexion is the skin's fine texture and:
   a) lack of sebum
   b) healthy color
   c) ability to resist organisms
   d) thick epidermis _____

4. The skin is thinnest on the:
   a) eyebrows
   b) eyelids
   c) forehead
   d) back of the hands _____

5. The skin is thickest on the:
   a) palms and soles
   b) abdomen
   c) buttocks
   d) thighs _____

6. The sudoriferous glands regulate:
   a) oil flow
   b) body temperature
   c) excess dryness
   d) emotional response _____

7. The outer protective layer of the skin is called the:
   a) dermis
   b) adipose
   c) epidermis
   d) reticular _____

8. No blood vessels are found in the:
   a) dermis
   b) eyelids
   c) subcutis
   d) epidermis
   _____

9. Blood vessels, nerves, and sweat and oil glands are found in the:
   a) epidermis
   b) dermis
   c) subcutaneous tissue
   d) scarf layer
   _____

10. The color of the skin depends on the blood supply to the skin and the coloring pigment called:
    a) keratin
    b) melanin
    c) lymph
    d) marrow
    _____

11. The layer of the epidermis that is continually being shed and replaced is the:
    a) stratum lucidum
    b) stratum corneum
    c) stratum granulosum
    d) stratum mucosum
    _____

12. The stratum corneum is also known as the:
    a) clear layer
    b) horny layer
    c) granular layer
    d) basal layer
    _____

13. Over a long period of time, continued pressure and friction on the skin will cause an area to become:
    a) slippery
    b) thinner
    c) callused
    d) scaly
    _____

14. The epidermis contains many:
    a) small nerve endings
    b) blood vessels
    c) adipose tissues
    d) small glands
    _____

15. Keratin is found in the:
    a) stratum mucosum
    b) stratum corneum
    c) stratum lucidum
    d) stratum granulosum
    _____

16. The outermost layer of the epidermis is the stratum:
    a) lucidum
    b) granulosum
    c) corneum
    d) germinativum
    _____

17. The stratum germinativum is also known as the:
    a) mucous layer   c) melanocyte layer
    b) basal layer   d) true skin   _____

18. The growth of the epidermis starts in the stratum:
    a) germinativum   c) corneum
    b) lucidum   d) granulosum   _____

19. The dermis is also known as the corium, cutis, derma, or:
    a) cuticle   c) subcutis
    b) true skin   d) cortex   _____

20. The reticular and papillary layers are found in the:
    a) Malpighian layer   c) scarf skin
    b) true skin   d) subcutis   _____

21. The papillary layer of the dermis contains looped capillaries and:
    a) adipose tissue   c) subcutaneous tissue
    b) arrector pili muscles d) tactile corpuscles _____

22. The reticular layer contains:
    a) granular cells   c) melanin
    b) tactile corpuscles   d) hair follicles   _____

23. Subcutaneous tissue consists mainly of:
    a) muscle tissue   c) keratin
    b) fatty cells   d) pigment   _____

24. Sensory nerve fibers in the skin react to:
    a) light   c) cold
    b) sound   d) fear   _____

25. Melanin is found in the stratum germinativum and:
    a) stratum corneum   c) papillary layer
    b) adipose tissue   d) reticular layer   _____

26. Melanin protects the skin from the harmful action of:
    a) bacteria   c) ultraviolet rays
    b) pressure   d) heat   _____

27. Skin elasticity is due to the presence of elastic tissue in the:
    a) dermis
    c) stratum lucidum
    b) stratum corneum
    d) stratum granulosum
    _____

28. The sebaceous glands secrete:
    a) blackheads
    c) oil
    b) salt
    d) perspiration
    _____

29. The function of sebum is to:
    a) minimize calluses
    c) promote new skin growth
    b) lubricate the skin
    d) excrete perspiration
    _____

30. Motor nerve fibers:
    a) excrete perspiration
    c) react to heat
    b) cause gooseflesh
    d) control the flow of sebum
    _____

31. The duct of an oil gland empties into the:
    a) blood stream
    c) sweat pore
    b) hair follicle
    d) fundus
    _____

32. No oil glands are found on the:
    a) palms
    c) forehead
    b) face
    d) scalp
    _____

33. The sudoriferous glands excrete:
    a) sebum
    c) odor
    b) perspiration
    d) bacteria
    _____

34. The two main divisions of the skin are the:
    a) reticular and papillary
    c) epidermis and scarf skin
    b) epidermis and dermis
    d) adipose and subcutaneous
    _____

35. The small openings of the sweat glands on the skin are called:
    a) follicles
    c) pores
    b) fundus
    d) ducts
    _____

36. The sweat and oil glands are known as:
    a) ductless glands
    c) duct glands
    b) endocrine glands
    d) sensory glands
    _____

37. The excretion of perspiration from the skin is under the control
of the:
   a) muscular system   c) endocrine system
   b) circulatory system   d) nervous system   _____

38. The blood and sweat glands of the skin regulate body heat by
maintaining a Fahrenheit temperature of about:
   a) 86.9°   c) 93.5°
   b) 96.8°   d) 98.6°   _____

39. The palms, soles, forehead, and armpits contain an abundance of:
   a) hair follicles   c) sudoriferous glands
   b) sebaceous glands   d) pores   _____

40. Endings of nerve fibers in the papillary layer are called:
   a) capillaries   c) tactile corpuscles
   b) papillae   d) lymph vessels   _____

41. The ability of the skin to stretch and regain its natural shape
reveals its:
   a) porosity   c) texture
   b) oiliness   d) pliability   _____

42. The subcutaneous tissue is:
   a) above the cuticle   c) below the dermis
   b) above the epidermis   d) below the adipose   _____

43. Motor nerve fibers are distributed to the:
   a) sweat glands   c) capillaries
   b) oil glands   d) arrector pili muscles   _____

44. Appendages of the skin include hair, nails, and:
   a) hair follicles   c) arrector pili muscles
   b) sweat and oil glands   d) sebum   _____

45. The skin is nourished by:
   a) sebum   c) melanin
   b) blood and lymph   d) keratin   _____

46. The study of the structure, functions, and disorders of the skin is known as:
    a) trichology
    b) etiology
    c) pathology
    d) dermatology
    _____

47. The study of the cause of a disease is:
    a) dermatology
    b) pathology
    c) etiology
    d) trichology
    _____

48. Pathology deals with the study of:
    a) the skin
    b) the hair
    c) disease
    d) the cause of disease
    _____

49. The foretelling of a probable course of a disease is known as:
    a) diagnosis
    b) prognosis
    c) recognition
    d) analysis
    _____

50. If a client has a skin disease, the cosmetologist should:
    a) prescribe treatment
    b) wear gloves
    c) refer the client to a physician
    d) suggest self-treatments
    _____

51. Itching is an example of a/an:
    a) subjective symptom
    b) objective symptom
    c) primary disorder
    d) secondary disorder
    _____

52. A papule is a:
    a) secondary skin lesion
    b) primary skin lesion
    c) subjective symptom
    d) objective symptom
    _____

53. Pus is most likely to be found in:
    a) vesicles
    b) leucoderma
    c) macules
    d) pustules
    _____

54. Another name for a vesicle is a/an:
    a) cicatrix
    b) abrasion
    c) blister
    d) scab
    _____

55. The skin lesion found in chapped lips and hands is a:
    a) fissure
    b) papule
    c) stain
    d) tumor
    _____

56. After a wound heals, a _____ may develop.
   a) vesicle   c) carbuncle
   b) cicatrix   d) furuncle   _____

57. An abnormal cell mass is known as a:
   a) papule   c) tumor
   b) macule   d) pustule   _____

58. A disease lasting a long time is described as:
   a) chronic   c) systemic
   b) acute   d) occupational   _____

59. A disease lasting a short time is described as:
   a) acute   c) congenital
   b) chronic   d) occupational   _____

60. An example of a seasonal disease is:
   a) dermatitis   c) ringworm
   b) smallpox   d) eczema   _____

61. A disease that spreads by personal contact is known as a/an:
   a) congenital disease   c) contagious disease
   b) systemic disease   d) occupational disease   _____

62. A disease that attacks a large number of people in a particular
    location is known as an:
   a) infectious disease   c) epidemic
   b) acute disease   d) allergy   _____

63. *Comedone* is the technical name for a:
   a) whitehead   c) blackhead
   b) macule   d) naevus   _____

64. *Milia* is the technical name for:
   a) whiteheads   c) pimples
   b) blackheads   d) naevus   _____

65. Acne, or a common pimple, is known as acne simplex or acne:
   a) rosacea   c) vulgaris
   b) comedone   d) singularis   _____

66. One of the symptoms of asteatosis is:
    a) oily skin
    c) dry skin
    b) a clear blister
    d) a fever blister _____

67. In seborrhea, the appearance of the skin is:
    a) dry and dull
    c) oily and shiny
    b) smooth and pink
    d) red and blotchy _____

68. Acne is indicated on the face by the presence of:
    a) steatomas
    c) carbuncles
    b) pimples
    d) dry scales _____

69. A steatoma may appear on the:
    a) face
    c) legs
    b) arms
    d) scalp _____

70. *Bromidrosis* means:
    a) lack of perspiration
    c) lack of sebum
    b) foul-smelling perspiration
    d) excess sebum _____

71. Excessive perspiration is:
    a) anhidrosis
    c) hyperhidrosis
    b) osmidrosis
    d) bromidrosis _____

72. *Anhidrosis* means:
    a) lack of perspiration
    c) foul-smelling perspiration
    b) excessive perspiration
    d) normal perspiration _____

73. People exposed to excessive heat may develop a condition known as:
    a) anhidrosis
    c) bromidrosis
    b) miliaria rubra
    d) eczema _____

74. The common term for lentigines is:
    a) birthmarks
    c) warts
    b) freckles
    d) calluses _____

75. Hyperhidrosis occurs most frequently in the area of the:
    a) elbows
    c) ankles
    b) armpits
    d) wrists _____

76. Eyelid surgery is:
    a) rhytidectomy
    b) blepharoplasty
    c) rhinoplasty
    d) mentoplasty _____

77. Certain chemicals found in cosmetics may cause:
    a) dermatitis simplex
    b) dermatitis venenata
    c) occupational simplex
    d) simplex venenata _____

78. Patches of dry, white scales on the scalp or skin may indicate the presence of:
    a) psoriasis
    b) eczema
    c) dermatitis
    d) seborrhea _____

79. Herpes simplex usually occurs around the:
    a) scalp
    b) ears
    c) forehead
    d) lips _____

80. A chronic inflammatory congestion of the cheeks and nose characterized by redness and dilation of the blood vessels is called:
    a) milia
    b) asteatosis
    c) seborrhea
    d) rosacea _____

81. Liver spots are known as:
    a) naevus
    b) leucoderma
    c) chloasma
    d) plasma _____

82. A birthmark is known as:
    a) albinism
    b) naevus
    c) leucoderma
    d) chloasma _____

83. Abnormal white patches on the skin are called:
    a) chloasma
    b) albinism
    c) leucoderma
    d) rosacea _____

84. *Miliaria rubra* is commonly known as:
    a) body odor
    b) prickly heat
    c) dermatitis
    d) acne simplex _____

85. Continued friction of the hands and feet may result in the formation of a:
   a) naevus
   b) tumor
   c) keratoma
   d) verruca
   _____

86. The technical term for *wart* is:
   a) keratoma
   b) papule
   c) verruca
   d) naevus
   _____

87. *Keratoma* is the technical term for a:
   a) callus
   b) wart
   c) tumor
   d) birthmark
   _____

88. The technique used to smooth scarred skin by sanding is known as:
   a) chemical peeling
   b) rhinoplasty
   c) blepharoplasty
   d) dermabrasion
   _____

89. A structural change in the skin tissues caused by injury or disease is a:
   a) fissure
   b) lesion
   c) infection
   d) wheal
   _____

90. Fatal skin cancer that starts with a mole is known as:
   a) melanotic tumor
   b) keratoma
   c) melanotic sarcoma
   d) vitiligo
   _____

Removing Unwanted Hair

1. The method used for permanent hair removal is:
   a) tweezing
   b) shaving
   c) depilatory
   d) electrolysis
   _____

2. An excessive growth of hair is called:
   a) canities
   b) monilethrix
   c) hypertrichosis
   d) trichoptilosis
   _____

3. The known causes of superfluous hair are hormonal imbalances, drugs, and:
   a) heredity
   b) alcohol use
   c) race
   d) diet
   _____

4. The shortwave method of electrolysis uses:
   a) a triple needle
   b) a single needle
   c) a double needle
   d) no needles
   _____

5. The galvanic method decomposes the hair:
   a) papilla
   b) follicle
   c) arrector pili
   d) shaft
   _____

6. One area that should *never* receive an electrolysis treatment is the:
   a) chin
   b) inner nose
   c) upper arm
   d) legs
   _____

7. The needle should be inserted into the hair follicle:
   a) at the opposite angle of hair growth
   b) straight down
   c) at the same angle as the hair growth
   d) at a 45-degree angle
   _____

8. Most depilatories:
   a) are used with machines
   b) have an alkaline pH
   c) destroy the papilla
   d) should not be used on oily skin
   _____

9. Waxing may cause hair to grow stronger because it:
   a) enlarges the hair root
   b) increases the blood supply to the hair follicle
   c) swells the hair shaft
   d) enlarges the hair follicle
   _____

10. A chemical depilatory is generally used on the:
    a) eyebrows
    b) underarms
    c) upper lip
    d) legs
    _____

11. After the removal of a wax depilatory, apply an emollient cream or a/an:
    a) talcum powder
    b) massage cream
    c) mineral oil
    d) antiseptic lotion
    _____

12. Shaved hair feels thicker because:
    a) the skin is contracted
    b) the follicle shrinks
    c) the hair ends are blunt
    d) the hair root is enlarged
    _____

13. Cold wax is removed from the treatment area with:
    a) tweezers
    b) solvent
    c) cotton cloth
    d) gloves
    _____

14. For those clients who cannot tolerate hot wax, another method available for the temporary removal of superfluous hair is:
    a) cold wax
    b) electrolysis
    c) thermolysis
    d) shortwave epilation
    _____

15. Wax must never be applied over warts, moles, growths, or abrasions because it may cause a/an:
    a) allergy
    b) ingrown hair
    c) irritation
    d) tumor
    _____

16. The temperature of hot wax should be tested on:
    a) the client's wrist
    b) your fingertip
    c) wax paper
    d) your arm
    _____

17. During a skin test, a depilatory must remain on the skin:
    a) 2–5 minutes
    b) 4–6 minutes
    c) 1–3 minutes
    d) 7–10 minutes
    _____

18. The most critical technique in electrolysis is:
    a) tweezer manipulation
    b) insertion
    c) the use of the foot pedal
    d) extraction
    _____

19. The cotton cloth is removed after a waxing treatment:
    a) in the direction of hair growth
    b) with tweezers
    c) in the opposite direction of hair growth
    d) slowly
    _____

20. If vellus hair is removed with hot wax, the skin may:
    a) lose its softness
    b) produce more follicles
    c) lose its elasticity
    d) produce coarser hair
    _____

Cells, Anatomy, and Physiology

1. Protoplasm is enclosed by the:
   a) centrosome
   b) cell membrane
   c) nucleolus
   d) nucleus
   _____

2. The protective covering on the mucous membranes is known as:
   a) epithelial tissue
   b) muscular tissue
   c) liquid tissue
   d) connective tissue
   _A_

3. Food materials for cellular growth and self-repair are found in the:
   a) nucleus
   b) cell matrix
   c) cytoplasm
   d) centrosome
   _C_

4. The nucleus of the cell controls:
   a) growth
   b) self-repair
   c) secretions
   d) reproduction
   _D_

5. The maintenance of normal, internal stability of an organism is known as:
   a) homeostasis
   b) mitosis
   c) metabolism
   d) anabolism
   _A_

6. Metabolism consists of two phases, anabolism and:
   a) mitosis
   b) homeostasis
   c) amitosis
   d) catabolism
   _D_

7. Body cells grow and reproduce during:
   a) anabolism
   b) catabolism
   c) mitosis
   d) amitosis
   _A_

8. The energy needed for muscular effort is released during:
   a) mitosis
   b) amitosis
   c) anabolism
   d) catabolism
   _____

9. Tissue is a group of similar:
   a) hormones
   b) muscles
   c) connections
   d) cells
   D

10. The heart, lungs, kidneys, stomach, and intestines are body:
    a) systems
    b) tissues
    c) organs
    d) functions
    C

11. Groups of organs that carry out a life activity of the body are:
    a) tissues
    b) systems
    c) muscles
    d) glands
    B

12. The integumentary system includes:
    a) the framework of the body
    b) the support of the skeleton
    c) the protective covering of the body
    d) the movements of the body
    _____

13. The skeletal system is important because it:
    a) covers and shapes the body
    b) supplies the body with blood
    c) is the physical foundation of the body
    d) carries nerve messages
    _____

14. Bone is composed of mainly calcium carbonate, calcium phosphate, and:
    a) 2/3 mineral matter
    b) 1/3 animal matter
    c) 2/3 animal matter
    d) 1/3 mineral matter
    _____

15. One of the functions of the bones is to:
    a) add weight to the body
    b) protect muscles
    c) give shape and support to the body
    d) house nerve endings
    _____

16. The scientific study of the bones, their structure, and their functions is called:
    a) osteology
    b) trichology
    c) myology
    d) biology
    _____

17. The portion of the skull that protects the brain is the:
    a) mandible   c) maxilla
    b) cranium   d) mastoid   *B*

18. An important function of bones is to:
    a) stimulate blood circulation   c) stimulate the muscles
    b) protect the organs   d) create calcium   _____

19. The shoulder girdle consists of one clavicle and:
    a) one scapula   c) one ulna
    b) one humerus   d) the ribs   _____

20. The cranial bones that are not affected by massage are the
    sphenoid and the:
    a) occipital   c) temporal
    b) ethmoid   d) frontal   _____

21. The small, fragile bones located at the front part of the inner wall
    of the eye sockets are the:
    a) nasal bones   c) lacrimal bones
    b) zygomatic bones   d) maxillae bones   _____

22. The largest and strongest bone of the face is the:
    a) lacrimal   c) mandible
    b) maxilla   d) zygomatic   _____

23. The place of union or junction of two or more bones is called a:
    a) ligament   c) vertebrae
    b) socket   d) joint   _____

24. The technical term for bone is:
    a) os   c) osteology
    b) orthopedic   d) integumentary   _____

25. The occipital bone forms the back and base of the:
    a) neck   c) chin
    b) cranium   d) forehead   _____

26. The parietal bones form the top and sides of the:
    a) face   c) cheeks
    b) cranium   d) neck   _____

27. The frontal bone forms the:
    a) upper jaw
    b) lower jaw
    c) forehead
    d) cheek
    _____

28. The temporal bones form the:
    a) forehead
    b) lower jaw
    c) eye sockets
    d) sides of the head
    _____

29. The ethmoid bone is situated:
    a) at the temple
    b) at the side of the cranium
    c) between the eye sockets
    d) on top of the cranium
    _____

30. The nasal bones form the:
    a) tip of the nose
    b) back of the nose
    c) bridge of the nose
    d) inner walls of the nose
    _____

31. The zygomatic or malar bones form the:
    a) outer walls of the nose
    b) cheeks
    c) mouth
    d) U-shaped bone in the throat
    _____

32. Maxillae are bones that form the:
    a) lower jaw
    b) upper jaw
    c) eye socket
    d) forehead
    _____

33. The mandible bone forms the:
    a) lower jaw
    b) upper jaw
    c) cheek
    d) nose
    _____

34. The cervical vertebrae form the:
    a) upper part of the spinal column
    b) protective framework for the chest
    c) U-shaped bone in the throat
    d) breastbone
    _____

35. The sphenoid bone joins together all bones of the:
    a) nose
    b) cranium
    c) ear
    d) neck
    _____

36. One of the functions of the muscular system is to:
    a) circulate the blood   c) produce body movements
    b) nourish the body   d) produce marrow   _____

37. The more fixed attachment of a muscle is called:
    a) the origin   c) the belly
    b) the insertion   d) ligament   _____

38. The more movable attachment of a muscle is called:
    a) the origin   c) ligament
    b) the insertion   d) the belly   _____

39. Muscles controlled by the will are called:
    a) involuntary muscles   c) reflex muscles
    b) voluntary muscles   d) nonstriated muscles   _____

40. The study of the structure, functions, and diseases of the muscles
    is called:
    a) cardiology   c) myology
    b) neurology   d) osteology   _____

41. In massage, pressure is usually directed on the muscles from the:
    a) insertion to orlgin   c) ligament to insertion
    b) origin to insertion   d) fixed attachment to the
                                       movable   _____

42. For its activities, the muscular system is dependent upon the
    skeletal system and the:
    a) lymphatic system   c) nervous system
    b) digestive system   d) circulatory system   _____

43. The muscles cover, shape, and support the:
    a) skeletal system   c) integumentary system
    b) nervous system   d) digestive system   _____

44. The epicranius muscle covers the:
    a) side of the head   c) bottom of the skull
    b) top of the skull   d) cheekbone   _____

45. The orbicularis oculi is a muscle that surrounds the margin of the:
   a) mouth   c) eye socket
   b) nose   d) head   _____

46. The corrugator extends along the:
   a) side of the nose   c) front of the ear
   b) eyebrow line   d) side of the cheek   _____

47. The procerus is a muscle of the:
   a) nose   c) ear
   b) eye   d) mouth   _____

48. The back part of the epicranius muscle is the:
   a) aponeurosis   c) frontalis
   b) occipitalis   d) corrugator   _____

49. The quadratus labii superioris is the muscle that raises the:
   a) ear   c) upper lip
   b) eye   d) lower lip   _____

50. The quadratus labii inferioris is the muscle that raises the:
   a) upper lip   c) eyebrow
   b) eyelid   d) lower lip   _____

51. The orbicularis oris:
   a) is responsible for snarling   c) compresses cheeks for
                                        blowing
   b) allows the lips to pucker   d) elevates the nostrils   _____

52. The mentalis is a muscle located in the:
   a) upper lip   c) jaw
   b) eyelid   d) chin   _____

53. The muscle that rotates the shoulder blades and controls the swinging movement of the arm is the:
   a) serratus anterior   c) trapezius
   b) deltoid   d) extensor   _____

54. The sternocleidomastoid muscle:
    a) flares the nostrils   c) depresses the lower jaw
    b) closes the lips   d) rotates the head   _____

55. The muscle responsible for turning the hand outward and palm upward is the:
    a) pronator   c) supinator
    b) flexor   d) extensor   _____

56. The nervous system controls and coordinates all body:
    a) structures   c) diseases
    b) functions   d) systems   _____

57. The central nervous system is composed of the brain and:
    a) spinal cord   c) heart
    b) sympathetic nerves   d) parasympathetic nerves   _____

58. A neuron is a/an:
    a) axon   c) axon terminal
    b) nerve cell   d) dendrite   _____

59. Touch, cold, heat, sight, and hearing are signaled to the brain by:
    a) reflexes   c) motor nerves
    b) afferent nerves   d) efferent nerves   _____

60. The motor nerves carry nerve impulses from the:
    a) sense organ to the brain   c) muscles to the brain
    b) brain to the muscles   d) skin to the brain   _____

61. The main divisions of the nervous system are the autonomic system, the peripheral system, and the:
    a) sympathetic system   c) spinal cord
    b) parasympathetic system   d) cerebrospinal system   _____

62. The muscles of the neck and back are affected by the:
    a) fifth nerve   c) eleventh nerve
    b) seventh nerve   d) thirteenth nerve   _____

63. The trigeminal is the chief sensory nerve of the:
    a) arm   c) chest
    b) face   d) shoulder   _____

64. The skin of the forehead and eyebrows is affected by the:
    a) supraorbital nerve
    b) infraorbital nerve
    c) supratrochlear nerve
    d) infratrochlear nerve _____

65. The skin of the lower lip and chin is affected by the:
    a) infraorbital nerve
    b) supraorbital nerve
    c) mental nerve
    d) auriculotemporal nerve _____

66. The skin of the upper lip and side of the nose is affected by the:
    a) infraorbital nerve
    b) supraorbital nerve
    c) zygomatic nerve
    d) auriculotemporal nerve _____

67. The seventh cranial nerve is also known as the:
    a) facial nerve
    b) trifacial nerve
    c) trigeminal nerve
    d) cervical nerve _____

68. The seventh cranial nerve is the chief motor nerve of the:
    a) arm
    b) chest
    c) face
    d) shoulder _____

69. The zygomatic motor nerve affects the muscles of the upper part of the:
    a) mouth
    b) cheek
    c) chin
    d) nose _____

70. The temporal nerve affects the muscles of the forehead, temple, and:
    a) nose
    b) upper lip
    c) ear
    d) eyebrow _____

71. Most of the muscles in the mouth are affected by the:
    a) mandibular nerve
    b) zygomatic nerve
    c) buccal nerve
    d) cervical nerve _____

72. The blood-vascular system comprises the heart, arteries, veins, and:
    a) lymph nodes
    b) adipose tissue
    c) duct glands
    d) capillaries _____

73. The upper heart chambers are called:
    a) ventricles
    c) valves
    b) atria
    d) pericardia
    _____

74. The lower heart chambers are called:
    a) ventricles
    c) valves
    b) vena cavas
    d) atria
    _____

75. Vessels that carry blood away from the heart are called:
    a) veins
    c) arteries
    b) capillaries
    d) valves
    _____

76. Vessels that carry blood to the heart are called:
    a) veins
    c) arteries
    b) capillaries
    d) aortas
    _____

77. The fluid part of the blood is called:
    a) plasma
    c) platelets
    b) corpuscles
    d) thrombocytes
    _____

78. Blood cells carrying oxygen to the cells are called:
    a) white corpuscles
    c) red corpuscles
    b) blood platelets
    d) hemoglobin
    _____

79. Blood cells that fight harmful bacteria are called:
    a) platelets
    c) red corpuscles
    b) leucocytes
    d) lacteals
    _____

80. The purpose of lymph nodes is to:
    a) equalize body temperature
    c) detoxify plasma
    b) regulate waste excretion
    d) detoxify lymph
    _____

81. The common carotid artery is located at the side of the:
    a) head
    c) neck
    b) face
    d) mouth
    _____

82. Blood reaches the nose through the:
    a) angular artery
    c) superior labial artery
    b) inferior labial artery
    d) submental artery
    _____

83. Blood is supplied to the lower region of the face by the:
    a) occipital artery
    b) external maxillary artery
    c) posterior artery
    d) frontal artery   _____

84. The parietal artery supplies blood to the:
    a) forehead
    b) back of the head
    c) crown and side of the head
    d) temples   _____

85. The inferior labial artery supplies blood to the:
    a) lower lip
    b) upper lip
    c) nose
    d) cheek   _____

86. The submental artery supplies blood to the:
    a) chin
    b) upper lip
    c) nose
    d) ear   _____

87. Blood is supplied to the brain, eye sockets, eyelids, and
    forehead by the:
    a) occipital artery
    b) supraorbital artery
    c) infraorbital artery
    d) posterior auricular artery   _____

88. The occipital artery supplies blood to the region of the:
    a) back of the head
    b) mouth and nose
    c) front of the head
    d) cheeks   _____

89. The palm of the hand contains:
    a) 8 carpal bones
    b) 5 metacarpal bones
    c) 10 phalanges
    d) 6 dorsal bones   _____

90. The ulna is a large bone of the:
    a) wrist
    b) hand
    c) upper arm
    d) forearm   _____

91. The wrist bones are called the:
    a) carpal bones
    b) metacarpal bones
    c) digital bones
    d) radial bones   _____

92. The longest and largest bone of the arm is the:
    a) ulna
    b) radius
    c) humerus
    d) clavicle   _____

93. The function of the extensor muscles is to:
    a) straighten the hands and fingers
    b) rotate the wrist
    c) close the hands and fingers
    d) separate the fingers _____

94. The function of the flexor muscles is to:
    a) open the hands and fingers
    b) bend the wrists
    c) rotate the hands and fingers
    d) close the fingers _____

95. The fingers of the hand are separated by movement of the:
    a) abductor muscles
    b) adductor muscles
    c) flexor muscles
    d) extensor muscles _____

96. The ulnar nerve supplies the:
    a) thumb side of the arm
    b) little finger side of the arm
    c) back of the hand
    d) top side of the fingers _____

97. The radial nerve supplies the:
    a) little finger side of the arm
    b) palm of the hand
    c) thumb side of the arm
    d) back of the hand _____

98. The digital nerves supply the:
    a) upper arm
    b) forearm
    c) back of the wrist
    d) fingers _____

99. The liver:
    a) excretes urine
    b) expells carbon dioxide
    c) discharges bile
    d) evacuates decomposed food _____

100. Nose breathing is healthier than mouth breathing because:
    a) more germs may live in saliva
    b) bacteria may be trapped in mucous membranes
    c) the throat may become irritated
    d) bacteria may infect the throat _____

Electricity and Light Therapy

1. Electricity produces chemical, magnetic, and:
   a) impulse effects
   b) rapid effects
   c) bactericidal effects
   d) heat effects _____

2. A substance that readily transmits electric current is a/an:
   a) conductor
   b) nonconductor
   c) insulator
   d) converter _____

3. The Tesla current is commonly called the:
   a) ultraviolet ray
   b) violet ray
   c) low-frequency current
   d) infrared ray _____

4. Rubber and silk are:
   a) conductors
   b) insulators
   c) electrodes
   d) converters _____

5. A metal such as copper wire is a/an:
   a) nonconductor
   b) conductor
   c) insulator
   d) converter _____

6. A constant electrical current flowing in one direction is called a/an:
   a) alternating current
   b) direct current
   c) faradic current
   d) steady current _____

7. A constant and direct current used to produce chemical effects on the tissues and fluids of the body is the:
   a) faradic current
   b) sinusoidal current
   c) Tesla current
   d) galvanic current _____

8. The apparatus that conducts electric current from a machine to the client's skin is a/an:
   a) modality
   b) insulator
   c) electrode
   d) wall plate

   _602_ ____

9. An alternating and interrupted current used principally to cause muscular contractions is the:
   a) faradic current
   b) high-frequency current
   c) Tesla current
   d) galvanic current

   _604_ ____

10. A unit of electrical pressure is referred to as a/an:
    a) ampere
    b) volt
    c) ohm
    d) watt

    _599_ ____

11. An ampere is a unit of electrical:
    a) usage
    b) resistance
    c) tension
    d) strength

    ____

12. An ohm is a unit of electrical:
    a) strength
    b) usage
    c) resistance
    d) tension

    _599_ ____

13. A 1/1000 part of an ampere is called a:
    a) volt
    b) kilowatt
    c) watt
    d) milliampere

    _599_ ____

14. The high-frequency current commonly used in the salon is the: → violet ray
    a) galvanic
    b) faradic
    c) Tesla
    d) sinusoidal

    ____

15. A substance that resists the passage of an electric current is a/an:
    a) insulator
    b) conductor
    c) converter
    d) rectifier

    _598_ ____

16. An electrical current used for its heat-producing effects is the:
    a) galvanic
    b) faradic
    c) high-frequency
    d) sinusoidal

    _606_ ____

17. A glass electrode that gives off sparks operates on: _606_
    a) galvanic current
    b) faradic current
    c) sinusoidal current
    d) high-frequency current

    ____

129

18. For a stimulating effect, the high-frequency electrode is:
    a) slightly lifted from the skin by the cosmetologist
    b) wrapped in astringent-soaked cotton
    c) kept in close contact with the skin
    d) wrapped in water-soaked cotton

19. The vibrator is an electrical appliance that:
    a) reduces blood circulation
    b) relaxes the area being treated
    c) stimulates the area being treated
    d) firms the area being treated

20. Facial and scalp steamers may be used to:
    a) decrease blood circulation
    b) increase perspiration
    c) treat tinea
    d) contract skin tissue

21. Treatment with light rays is called:
    a) heat therapy
    b) light therapy
    c) electrotherapy
    d) ultraviolet treatment

22. About 80% of natural sunshine consists of:
    a) ultraviolet rays
    b) actinic rays
    c) visible light rays
    d) phoresis

23. The shortest and least penetrating light rays of the spectrum are the:
    a) infrared rays
    b) ultraviolet rays
    c) low-frequency rays
    d) white rays

24. The light rays of the spectrum that can produce the most heat are:
    a) ultraviolet rays
    b) actinic rays
    c) blue light rays
    d) infrared rays

25. Resistance to disease may be increased by limited exposure to:
    a) red light rays
    b) infrared rays
    c) white light rays
    d) ultraviolet rays

26. The skin can tan if it is exposed to:
    a) white dermal light
    b) red dermal light
    c) infrared rays
    d) ultraviolet rays

27. _____ rays destroy hair pigment.
    a) Infrared
    b) Ultraviolet
    c) White
    d) Visible

    _____

28. To receive the full benefit from ultraviolet rays, the area treated should be:
    a) coated with sunscreen
    b) damp
    c) moisturized
    d) bare

    _____

29. The combination light is the:
    a) blue light
    b) white light
    c) ultraviolet light
    d) red light

    _____

30. The average distance you should place an infrared lamp from the skin is about:
    a) 24"
    b) 10"
    c) 18"
    d) 30"

    _____

Chemistry

1. Organic chemistry is the study of all substances containing:
   a) carbon   c) organisms
   b) hydrogen   d) water   _____

2. Grass, gasoline, and antibiotics are examples of:
   a) inorganic substances   c) solid matter
   b) organic substances   d) liquid matter   _B_

3. Matter is anything that:
   a) is a solid or liquid   c) contains carbon
   b) is soluble in water   d) occupies space   _D_

4. Objects with a definite form are examples of:
   a) solids   c) gases
   b) elements   d) bases   _A_

5. The smallest particle of an element is the:
   a) atom   c) molecule
   b) nucleus   d) electron   _A_

6. The simplest form of matter that cannot be decomposed by chemical means is a/an:
   a) element   c) gas
   b) oxide   d) emulsion   _____

7. When two of the same atoms are joined, the result is a/an
   a) compound   c) element
   b) mixture   d) suspension   _C_

8. When two or more elements combine chemically in definite weight proportions, they form a:
   a) mixture
   b) compound
   c) suspension
   d) solution

   _____

9. Hydrogen peroxide is an example of a/an:
   a) salt
   b) acid
   c) alkali
   d) oxide

   _____

10. When the hydrogen in an acid is replaced by a metal, the result is a/an:
    a) alkali
    b) mixture
    c) salt
    d) oxide

    _____

11. Sodium chloride is an example of:
    a) an oxide
    b) an alkali
    c) a salt
    d) an acid

    _____

12. An alteration of the properties of a substance without the formation of any new substance is a:
    a) solution
    b) physical change
    c) compound
    d) chemical change

    _____

13. The most abundant element on earth is:
    a) oxygen
    b) hydrogen
    c) nitrogen
    d) ammonia

    _____

14. The second most abundant element known is:
    a) peroxide
    b) oxygen
    c) nitrogen
    d) hydrogen

    D

15. Pure water with a pH of 7 is considered to be:
    a) neutral
    b) acid
    c) alkaline
    d) mild

    A

16. Water is composed of:
    a) 2 volumes of hydrogen and 1 volume of oxygen
    b) 2 volumes of hydrogen and 2 volumes of oxygen
    c) 1 volume of hydrogen and 2 volumes of oxygen
    d) 1 volume of hydrogen and 1 volume of oxygen

    A

17. Removing impurities from water by passing it through a porous substance is the process of:
    a) distillation
    b) neutralization
    c) filtration
    d) oxidation
    _____

18. When ice melts and becomes water, it is a:
    a) chemical change
    b) physical change
    c) synthetic process
    d) chemical reaction
    _____

19. The ability of a substance to resist scratching refers to its:
    a) color
    b) hardness
    c) density
    d) specific gravity
    _____

20. Lighting a match or burning wood is an example of:
    a) slow oxidation
    b) light therapy
    c) reduction
    d) combustion
    _____

21. The pH of hair is:
    a) 2.5–3.5
    b) 3.5–4.5
    c) 4.5–5.5
    d) 7.0–8.5
    _C_

22. Dandruff shampoos may fall under the category of:
    a) amphoteric shampoos
    b) cationic shampoos
    c) anionic shampoos
    d) nonionic shampoos
    _____

23. Baby shampoos generally are classified as:
    a) ampholytes
    b) cationics
    c) anionics
    d) nonionics
    _____

24. The hydrophilic end of a shampoo molecule is attracted to:
    a) oil
    b) hair
    c) water
    d) conditioner
    _C_

25. Most conditioners fall in the pH range of:
    a) 4.0–7.5
    b) 3.5–6.0
    c) 2.0–8.0
    d) 7.0–9.0
    _B_

26. Temporary haircoloring contains:
    a) aniline derivatives
    b) developer
    c) ammonia
    d) certified colors
    _D_

27. A preparation made by dissolving a solid, liquid, or gaseous substance in another substance is a:
   a) suspension
   c) solution
   b) compound
   d) mixture _____

28. A liquid used to dissolve a substance is called the:
   a) solute
   c) solvent
   b) concentrate
   d) volatile substance _____

29. Solvents that mix easily are:
   a) immiscible
   c) emulsions
   b) miscible
   d) united with the aid of a gum _____

30. A semisolid mixture of an organic substance and a medicinal agent is a/an:
   a) soap
   c) ointment
   b) mucilage
   d) paste _____

31. Traditional soap is formed from the chemical combination of:
   a) an alkali and a fat
   c) a detergent and potassium
   b) an alkali and a salt
   d) a fat and alcohol _____

32. Witch hazel is a solution that works as a/an:
   a) astringent
   c) disinfectant
   b) skin softener
   d) protective cream _____

33. The purpose of a cold cream is to:
   a) eradicate wrinkles
   c) strengthen facial muscles
   b) cleanse skin
   d) decrease perspiration _____

34. An alkaline causes the hair to:
   a) harden and shrink
   c) stretch and return
   b) soften and swell
   d) close the cuticle layer _____

35. The classification of haircolor that does not lift natural melanin but requires 10 volume developer is:
   a) oxidative deposit-only
   c) nonoxidative permanent
   b) oxidative permanent
   d) semi-permanent _____

36. The product formulated to remove color buildup or stain from the cuticle is a:
    a) dye solvent
    b) protein color remover
    c) oil-based color remover
    d) liquid bleach _____

37. The lotion similar to a cleansing cream, but with less oil is:
    a) freshener lotion
    b) medicated lotion
    c) astringent lotion
    d) cleansing lotion _____

38. The eye makeup that contains wax and thickeners is:
    a) eye pencil
    b) mascara
    c) eye shadow
    d) eyeliner _____

39. Calamine lotion is an example of a/an:
    a) suspension
    b) ointment
    c) emulsion
    d) solution _____

40. Hydrogen peroxide may be found in:
    a) semi-permanent color
    b) sodium hydroxide relaxers
    c) ammonium thioglycolate solutions
    d) neutralizers _____

41. Quats may be included in moisturizers for their:
    a) ability to repel water
    b) ability to aid in rinsing
    c) ability to attach to hair fibers
    d) lubricating ability _____

42. When oxidative permanent color is applied to the hair, it creates a/an:
    a) alkaline reaction
    b) acid reaction
    c) physical change
    d) rapid combustion _____

43. The ingredient in deodorant soap that may increase skin sensitivity to sun is:
    a) phenol
    b) triclocarban
    c) glycerine
    d) fatty acids _____

44. The primary ingredient in lipstick is:
    a) castor oil
    b) mineral oil
    c) water
    d) beeswax _____

45. Hair sprays are mainly a combination of:
    a) polymers and perfume
    b) alcohol and water
    c) plasticizers and polymers
    d) aerosol and alcohol _____

The Salon Business

1. When selecting the location for a salon, you should consider:
   a) your personnel policies
   b) the number of staff to hire
   c) the services you will offer
   d) direct competition _____

2. An owner and/or salon manager should have a knowledge of general business principles and:
   a) psychology
   b) current fashion trends
   c) basic salon equipment repairs
   d) plumbing _____

3. Building maintenance and renovations are regulated by:
   a) federal laws
   b) local ordinances
   c) state laws
   d) the department of licensing _____

4. Information about which products are selling well and which items do not sell well can be seen in the salon's:
   a) consumption records
   b) inventory records
   c) service records
   d) petty cash book _____

5. The type of ownership that subjects the owner to the most limited personal loss is the:
   a) corporation
   b) co-ownership
   c) individual ownership
   d) partnership _____

6. Salon owners purchase insurance policies to protect themselves against suits for:
   a) increases in rent
   b) loss of employees
   c) malpractice
   d) decreases in clients _____

7. Major purchases of supplies should be made:
   a) after tax time
   b) when suppliers offer special prices
   c) before income taxes are filed
   d) when they are needed
   _____

8. In a well-organized beauty salon, the flow of clients is directed toward the:
   a) reception area
   b) shampooing area
   c) style stations
   d) parking area
   _____

9. For satisfactory service, it is essential that the salon have good plumbing and sufficient:
   a) office space
   b) lighting
   c) parking facilities
   d) public transportation
   _____

10. The best form of advertising is a:
    a) neon sign
    b) pleased client
    c) newspaper ad
    d) window display
    _____

11. Closer contact is made with potential clients by using:
    a) newspaper advertising
    b) radio advertising
    c) yellow pages advertising
    d) direct mail advertising
    _____

12. Salons can be located near each other if they have:
    a) a different type of clientele
    b) different retail products
    c) a different number of employees
    d) different payment options
    _____

13. Social Security is covered under:
    a) local laws
    b) state laws
    c) federal laws
    d) income tax laws
    _____

14. The largest expense item in operating a beauty salon is:
    a) rent
    b) salaries
    c) supplies
    d) advertising
    _____

15. The "quarterback" of the salon is the:
    a) manager
    b) stylist
    c) shampoo person
    d) receptionist
    _____

16. An accurate reflection of what is taking place in the salon at a given time can be seen in:
    a) a business plan
    b) yearly records
    c) the appointment book
    d) an income tax return   _____

17. Salon and individual licenses are covered by:
    a) federal laws
    b) county laws
    c) local laws
    d) state laws   _____

18. When booking appointments by telephone in the salon, you should:
    a) give most clients to the new cosmetologist
    b) be familiar with all services and products available
    c) give most clients to the established cosmetologist
    d) use a pencil in case of cancellations   _____

19. One requisite of a good telephone personality is:
    a) correct speech
    b) a pen and pad nearby
    c) bilingual skills
    d) a loud voice   _____

20. When purchasing an established salon, an investigation should be performed to determine:
    a) the current clients
    b) the last three owners
    c) any default in debt payment
    d) what the owner paid for the property   _____

21. A very important responsibility in salon operation is the handling of:
    a) lighting
    b) competitors
    c) appointments
    d) storage   _____

22. State laws usually cover:
    a) excise taxes
    b) licensure
    c) Social Security
    d) building codes   _____

23. When listening to a client's complaint, it is important to avoid:
    a) being sympathetic
    b) promising free service
    c) interrupting them
    d) apologizing   _____

24. In order to make selling more agreeable and productive, the cosmetologist must be:
   a) self-confident
   c) forceful
   b) aware of competition sales
   d) cautious _____

25. The first step in successful selling in the beauty salon is to:
   a) show the product's use
   c) sell yourself
   b) have a sale
   d) advertise _____

26. A salon owned by stockholders and which has a state charter is a/an:
   a) corporation
   c) partnership
   b) individual ownership
   d) joint ownership _____

27. Before selling a service or a product to a client, you must first determine if there is:
   a) sufficient income potential
   c) an upcoming sale
   b) a product guarantee
   d) a need for it _____

28. The approximate percent of a salon's income spent on salaries is:
   a) 25
   c) 50
   b) 35
   d) 75 _____

29. Client records should be kept:
   a) at your station
   c) in the dispensary
   b) in the office
   d) at a central location _____

30. If two people own a salon together, that type of ownership is a/an:
   a) individual ownership
   c) corporation
   b) chain salon
   d) partnership _____

31. Products that are sold to clients are:
   a) stock supplies
   c) consumption supplies
   b) retail supplies
   d) wholesale supplies _____

32. Local, state, and federal tax laws require a business to maintain:
   a) proper business records
   c) a dress code for employees
   b) the parking area
   d) an advertising budget _____

33. In order to maintain an accurate and efficient control of supplies, it is necessary to have an organized:
    a) inventory system
    b) purchase system
    c) security system
    d) service record   _____

34. Daily sales slips, appointment books, and petty cash books should be retained for at least:
    a) 7 months
    b) 7 years
    c) 6 months
    d) 6 years   _____

35. Payroll books and cancelled checks should be retained for:
    a) 7 months
    b) 7 years
    c) 6 months
    d) 6 years   _____

36. Federal laws cover:
    a) income tax
    b) renovations
    c) leases
    d) licenses   _____

37. Advertising should be concentrated around:
    a) your personal schedule
    b) newspaper schedules
    c) the holidays
    d) traditionally slow periods   _____

38. A salon phone should be answered:
    a) after two rings
    b) promptly
    c) when clients are not at the reception desk
    d) on the hour and every 15 minutes after   _____

39. When handling complaints by phone, you should:
    a) have the owner handle it
    b) suggest another salon
    c) allow the cosmetologist concerned to handle it
    d) use self-control and courtesy   _____

40. The most important step in selling is to:
    a) determine the client's needs
    b) only offer products that sell themselves
    c) offer a variety of inexpensive products
    d) advertise sales in advance   _____

Typical State Board Examination
Test 1: 100 Multiple-Choice Questions

DIRECTIONS: Carefully read each statement. Choose the word or phrase that correctly completes the meaning of each statement and write the corresponding letter on the line.

1. One of the major elements required for good health is proper:
   a) diet
   b) training
   c) clothing
   d) coworkers

   _A_

2. For a good sitting posture, keep your knees and:
   a) arms close together
   b) hips relaxed
   c) feet close together
   d) ankles crossed

   _C_

3. A successful cosmetologist is a skilled:
   a) storyteller
   b) listener
   c) fitness expert
   d) fashion expert

   _B_

4. Bacteria are not harmed by disinfectants while in the:
   a) vegetative stage
   b) spore-forming stage
   c) active stage
   d) mitosis stage

   _____

5. Bacilli are bacteria with a:
   a) corkscrew shape
   b) round shape
   c) rod shape
   d) curved shape

   _C_

6. Acquired immune deficiency syndrome (AIDS):
   a) is caused by needle use
   b) is a form of herpes
   c) attacks the nervous system
   d) is caused by the HIV virus

   _D_

7. Surfaces that may be sterilized are:
   a) skin
   b) nonporous
   c) nail plates
   d) wood and plastic

   _B_

8. Disinfection is one step below sterilization because it does not:
   a) kill microbes
   b) kill bacterial spores
   c) have an odor
   d) clean surfaces

   _____

9. A disinfectant that is "Formulated for Hospitals and Health Care Facilities" must be pseudomonacidal, bactericidal, fungicidal, and:
   a) pneumonicidal
   b) inexpensive
   c) virucidal
   d) easy to dilute for other services

   _____

10. Rather than using bar soaps, which can grow bacteria, you should provide:
    a) baby cleanser
    b) pump-type antibacterial soap
    c) alcohol wipes
    d) a washcloth

    _____

11. The technical term for eyelash hair is:
    a) barba
    b) cilia
    c) capilli
    d) supercilia

    _____

12. The chemical composition of hair varies with its:
    a) color
    b) length
    c) thickness
    d) growth pattern

    _____

13. The club-shaped structure that forms the lower part of the hair root is the:
    a) arrector pili
    b) bulb
    c) papilla
    d) hair shaft

    _____

14. The growing phase of hair is known as:
    a) anagen
    b) mitosis
    c) catagen
    d) telogen

    _____

15. A topical solution applied to the scalp that is medically proven to regrow hair is:
    a) finasteride
    b) astringent
    c) monoxidil
    d) hot oil

    _____

16. Long, thick pigmented hair is known as:
    a) barba
    b) terminal
    c) supercilia
    d) vellus

    _____

17. Hair flowing in the same direction is known as:
    a) the natural parting   c) a cowlick
    b) the hair stream   d) the hairline   _____

18. Wiry hair may have a hard, glassy finish caused by:
    a) raised cuticle scales   c) loss of pigment
    b) overconditioning   d) flat cuticle scales   _____

19. A miniaturization of certain scalp follicles contributes to:
    a) androgenetic alopecia   c) alopecia areata
    b) postpartum alopecia   d) telogen effluvium   _____

20. Trichoptilosis is the technical name for:
    a) beaded hair   c) gray hair
    b) split ends   d) ringed hair   _____

21. The medical term for dandruff is:
    a) pityriasis   c) tinea
    b) pediculosis   d) monilethrix   _____

22. A cape must not touch the client's skin because it may:
    a) be irritating to the client c) be damp
    b) have cut hair on it   d) be a carrier of disease _____

23. In order to determine the water temperature during a shampoo,:
    a) test it on your wrist   c) check with the client
                                       frequently
    b) keep one finger over the   d) keep the faucet set at one
       spray nozzle   temperature   _____

24. Proper shampooing helps prevent:
    a) split ends   c) a flexible scalp
    b) scalp disorders   d) pediculosis   _____

25. To maintain proper tension during haircutting,:
    a) saturate hair   c) do not cut past your
                                       second knuckle
    b) use a razor   d) allow your index and
                                       middle fingers to overlap _____

26. The amount of elevation from the head form is:
    a) dictated by parting size   c) measured in degrees
    b) equal to the subsection size   d) measured in inches   _____

27. Thinning is not advisable in the:
    a) parting and nape   c) hairline and guideline
    b) hairline and nape   d) parting and hairline   _____

28. The results of a high-elevation haircut should be:
    a) longer in the crown   c) one length
    b) the same length throughout   d) longer in the nape
       the head   _____

29. If the head is pushed forward during a haircut, the results will be:
    a) wispy   c) longer underneath
    b) closely tapered   d) undercut   _____

30. Transition lines in hairstyling are usually:
    a) horizontal   c) vertical
    b) curved   d) diagonal   _____

31. The actual surface quality of the hair is referred to as:
    a) density   c) texture
    b) volume   d) depth   _____

32. The place the eye sees first in a hairstyle is the point of:
    a) proportion   c) balance
    b) harmony   d) emphasis   _____

33. A tight, firm, long-lasting curl is produced by the:
    a) full-stem curl   c) half-stem curl
    b) no-stem curl   d) open center curl   _____

34. A finished curl is not affected by the:
    a) size of the curl   c) shape of the base
    b) amount of hair used   d) direction of the curl   _____

35. If hair is wound one complete turn around a roller, it will create:
    a) a C-shape   c) an explosion of curl
    b) a wave   d) ringlets   _____

36. When a smooth comb-out is desired, be sure to:
    a) use a large tooth comb   c) style with your fingers
    b) brush the hair smooth   d) brush hair ends only   _____

37. The temperature of heated thermal irons is tested on:
    a) a strand of hair   c) a piece of tissue paper
    b) a damp cloth   d) wax paper   _____

38. Before the hair is combed out after blow-dry styling, it should
    be thoroughly:
    a) smoothed   c) coated with gel
    b) heated   d) cooled   _____

39. The styling of hair with an air waver is performed in the same
    manner as:
    a) thermal waving   c) a chemical blow-out
    b) finger waving   d) blow-out waving   _____

40. Before perming, the hair should be tested for porosity and:
    a) density   c) elasticity
    b) length   d) texture   _____

41. The size of the curl or wave in permanent waving is controlled
    by:
    a) the size of the perm rod   c) processing time
    b) the solution used   d) the neutralization process _____

42. The diameter of the individual hair strand is the hair's:
    a) elasticity   c) porosity
    b) texture   d) density   _____

43. Average permanent wave partings should match:
    a) the size of the end papers c) from crown to nape
    b) the diameter of the rod   d) in width and length   _____

44. When a perm is activated by outside heat, such as a hood dryer,
    it is:
    a) endothermic   c) exothermic
    b) neutral balanced   d) external processing   _____

45. A weak or limp wave formation is the result of:
    a) using too much solution   c) tension winding
    b) underprocessing   d) incorrect blocking   _____

46. Acid-balanced and neutral permanent wave lotions produce:
    a) deep, tight waves   c) spiral curls
    b) shorter-lasting waves   d) soft, natural-looking waves   _____

47. A predisposition test is performed before a haircolor service to
    determine:
    a) haircolor results   c) processing time
    b) allergy to aniline   d) proper application method   _____

48. The lightest primary color is:
    a) yellow   c) red
    b) blue   d) white   _____

49. Orange is created by mixing:
    a) red and blue   c) yellow and blue
    b) red and white   d) yellow and red   _____

50. Semi-permanent color:
    a) requires an oxidizer   c) will fade without a regrowth
    b) is endothermic   d) lasts 4–6 weeks   _____

51. Dry peroxide is used to:
    a) thicken liquid color   c) dilute other strengths
    b) decrease processing time   d) boost peroxide strength   _____

52. Progressive haircolors fall under the classification of:
    a) vegetable tints   c) metallic dyes
    b) compound dyes   d) oxidative tints   _____

53. Non-ammonia alkali and a low volume developer is used with:
    a) oxidative deposit-only   c) polymer semi-permanent
       color   color
    b) traditional semi-permanent d) nonoxidative permanent
       color   color   _____

54. A disadvantage of cream peroxide is that it:
    a) may dry too quickly
    b) is hard to mix with bleach
    c) can become lumpy
    d) may dilute the color strength
    _____

55. To lighten previously tinted hair,:
    a) apply powder bleach
    b) use a higher volume of peroxide
    c) use a color remover before tinting
    d) select a lighter single-process tint
    _____

56. A factor that affects the processing time of a chemical relaxer is:
    a) the season of the year
    b) hair porosity
    c) previous styling products used
    d) hair length
    _____

57. The test that determines the hair's degree of elasticity is known as the:
    a) pull test
    b) match test
    c) strand test
    d) finger test
    _____

58. The two general types of hair relaxers are ammonium thioglycolate and:
    a) fillers
    b) sodium hydroxide
    c) pressing oil
    d) compound henna
    _____

59. If hair "beads" from the scalp during a relaxer,:
    a) rinse immediately
    b) mist with the water bottle
    c) add neutralizer
    d) continue to process
    _____

60. Hair pressing generally lasts:
    a) overnight
    b) until shampooed
    c) one week
    d) 4–6 weeks
    _____

61. When pressing gray hair, use light pressure and:
    a) more pressing oil
    b) moderate heat
    c) smaller subsections
    d) a larger pressing comb
    _____

62. A hard press in which a hot curling iron is passed through the hair first is called a:
    a) double press
    b) chemical press
    c) thermal press
    d) single press
    _____

63. A scalp may be classified as normal, flexible, or:
    a) brittle   c) porous
    b) thin   d) tight   _____

64. Each time a human hair wig is dry-cleaned, it should be:
    a) resized   c) reknotted
    b) reconditioned   d) restretched   _____

65. If a client is accidentally cut during a manicure, apply _____ to
    stop the bleeding.
    a) a styptic pencil   c) powdered alum
    b) petroleum jelly   d) alcohol   _____

66. While a manicure is performed, instruments should be kept in a:
    a) drawer   c) bead sterilizer
    b) jar sanitizer   d) plastic bag attached to
                                            station   _____

67. A hand massage may be given during a manicure:
    a) before polish   c) before filing
    b) before soaking   d) before pushing cuticles   _____

68. Brushes used for acrylic overlays are cleaned by dipping into:
    a) alcohol   c) a weak quat
    b) soapy water   d) polish remover   _____

69. The strongest material used for nail wrapping is:
    a) mending tissue   c) silk
    b) acrylic   d) linen   _____

70. Fungus is caused by the trapping of dirt and _____
    between artificial nail products and the natural nail.
    a) nail polish   c) moisture
    b) primer   d) natural oils   _____

71. The light color of the lunula is caused by light reflection where:
    a) the free edge and the nail   c) the matrix and cuticle join
       bed join
    b) the nail bed and walls join   d) the matrix and connective
                                            tissue of the nail bed join   _____

72. The technical name for the nail is:
    a) onyx
    c) onychosis
    b) onychauxis
    d) oncyhia
    _____

73. The medical term for brittle nails is:
    a) onychophagy
    c) onychorrhexis
    b) onychia
    d) onychocryptosis
    _____

74. Bitten nails are referred to as:
    a) onychophagy
    c) onychorrhexis
    b) onychia
    d) onychocryptosis
    _____

75. One area the cosmetologist is not licensed to massage is the:
    a) leg below the knee
    c) leg above the knee
    b) upper chest
    d) back of the leg
    _____

76. The most invigorating massage movement is:
    a) kneading
    c) friction
    b) tapotement
    d) vibration
    _____

77. Following the removal of blackheads, apply:
    a) a mud mask
    c) astringent
    b) massage cream
    d) cool towels
    _____

78. Studies show acne may be due to:
    a) lack of skin care
    c) chocolate
    b) fast foods
    d) hereditary factors
    _____

79. A household ingredient that may be used for a hydrating effect in a mask is:
    a) strawberries
    c) egg whites
    b) honey
    d) cucumbers
    _____

80. Eyebrows are properly tweezed:
    a) in an upward motion
    c) in the direction of their growth
    b) after foundation is applied
    d) after every makeup application
    _____

81. The layer of the epidermis that is continually being shed is the:
    a) stratum lucidum
    b) stratum corneum
    c) stratum granulosum
    d) stratum mucosum
    _____

82. The duct of an oil gland empties into the:
    a) hair follicle
    b) fundus
    c) blood stream
    d) sweat pore
    _____

83. *Comedone* is the technical name for a:
    a) macule
    b) blackhead
    c) whitehead
    d) naevus
    _____

84. In seborrhea, the appearance of the skin is:
    a) dry and dull
    b) smooth and pink
    c) oily and shiny
    d) red and blotchy
    _____

85. Hyperhidrosis occurs most frequently in the area of the:
    a) forehead
    b) bottom of the feet
    c) elbows
    d) armpits
    _____

86. The cotton cloth is removed after a wax treatment:
    a) with tweezers
    b) slowly
    c) in the direction of hair growth
    d) in the opposite direction of hair growth
    _____

87. The temperature of hot wax should be tested on:
    a) the client's wrist
    b) your fingertip
    c) your arm
    d) wax paper
    _____

88. The heart, lungs, kidneys, stomach, and intestines are body:
    a) systems
    b) organs
    c) functions
    d) tissues
    _____

89. One of the functions of the bones is to:
    a) give shape and support to the body
    b) add weight to the body
    c) house nerve endings
    d) protect muscles
    _____

90. A unit of electrical pressure is referred to as a/an:
    a) ampere   c) ohm
    b) volt   d) watt   _____

91. The Tesla current is commonly called the:
    a) ultraviolet ray   c) low-frequency current
    b) violet ray   d) infrared ray   _____

92. About 80% of natural sunshine consists of:
    a) ultraviolet rays   c) visible light rays
    b) actinic rays   d) infrared rays   _____

93. The smallest particle of an element is the:
    a) atom   c) molecule
    b) nucleus   d) electron   _____

94. Baby shampoos are generally classified as:
    a) amphoterics   c) anionics
    b) cationics   d) nonionics   _____

95. An alkaline causes the hair to:
    a) harden and shrink   c) stretch and return
    b) soften and swell   d) close the cuticle layer   _____

96. Quats may be included in moisturizers for their ability to:
    a) repel water   c) attach to hair fibers
    b) aid in rinsing   d) lubricate   _____

97. The ingredient in deodorant soap that may increase skin
    sensitivity to the sun is:
    a) phenol   c) triclocarbon
    b) glycerine   d) fatty acids   _____

98. Salon and individual licenses are covered by:
    a) federal laws   c) local laws
    b) county regulations   d) state laws   _____

99. Before selling a service or product to a client, you must first
    determine if there is:
    a) a need for it   c) sufficient income potential
    b) an upcoming sale   d) a product guarantee   _____

100. Payroll books and canceled checks should be retained for:
    a) 7 months
    b) 7 years
    c) 6 months
    d) 6 years   _____

Typical State Board Examination
Test 2: 100 Multiple-Choice Questions

DIRECTIONS: Carefully read each statement. Choose the word or phrase that correctly completes the meaning of each statement and write the corresponding letter on the line.

1. Public hygiene is also known as:
   a) personal grooming   c) sanitation
   b) sterilization   d) disinfection

   C

2. For a comfortable sitting posture, keep the soles of the feet:
   a) on the floor   c) extended
   b) crossed   d) elevated

   A

3. Proper conduct in relation to employer, clients, and coworkers is called professional:
   a) personality   c) courtesy
   b) ethics   d) honesty

   B

4. The inactive phase in the life cycle of bacteria is known as the:
   a) pathogenic stage   c) mitosis stage
   b) nonpathogenic stage   d) spore-forming stage

   D   *C*

5. An example of a general infection is a:
   a) boil   c) chapped lip
   b) syphilis   d) keratoma

   A   *B*

6. AIDS is caused by:
   a) lack of proper nutrition c) the HIV virus
   b) herpes   d) unsanitary habits

   C

155

7. The level of decontamination not required in the salon is:
   a) sanitation
   b) sterilization
   c) decontamination
   d) cleaning

   _B_

8. If a salon implement comes into contact with blood or bodily fluids, it should be cleaned and completely immersed in:
   a) alcohol
   b) an EPA-registered disinfectant
   c) an OSHA-registered antiseptic
   d) formalin

   _C_

9. Two elements of universal precautions involve your personal hygiene and:
   a) your health
   b) your attitude
   c) your personal appearance
   d) salon cleanliness

   _A_

10. The study of the hair is:
    a) pathology
    b) dermatology
    c) trichology
    d) etiology

    _C_

11. The papilla fits into the:
    a) medulla
    b) root
    c) bulb
    d) hair shaft

    _C_

12. Hair pigment is found in the:
    a) cuticle
    b) cortex
    c) medulla
    d) follicle

    _A_

13. Vellus hair is:
    a) pigmented
    b) nonpigmented
    c) coarse
    d) curly

    _C_

14. The resting phase of the hair growth cycle is known as:
    a) anagen
    b) catagen
    c) biogen
    d) telogen

    _D_

15. The ability of hair to absorb moisture is its:
    a) texture
    b) elasticity
    c) density
    d) porosity

    _D_

65

16. Androgenetic alopecia:
    a) alters follicle structure
    b) does not alter the number of follicles
    c) does not change follicle size
    d) increases the number of follicles

17. The cosmetologist may recognize miniaturized hairs on a client's scalp by their:
    a) flat ends
    b) round ends
    c) split ends
    d) pointy ends

18. An abnormal development of hair is known as:
    a) hypertrichosis
    b) trichorrhexis nodosa
    c) trichoptilosis
    d) hyperhidrosis

19. A prescription pill for the treatment of androgenetic alopecia is:
    a) monoxidil
    b) follicidil
    c) finasteride
    d) methacrylate

20. The medical term for ringworm is:
    a) pediculosis
    b) tinea
    c) pityriasis
    d) scutula

21. A furuncle is commonly known as a:
    a) wart
    b) cold sore
    c) follicle infection
    d) boil

22. When draping, a neck strip or towel is necessary to prevent the client's skin from:
    a) feeling uncomfortable
    b) touching the cape
    c) getting wet
    d) sticking to cut hair ends

23. Thorough brushing of the scalp should not be given before a:
    a) haircolor
    b) shampoo
    c) haircut
    d) scalp treatment

24. Medicated shampoos will affect:
    a) the style results
    b) the conditioner process
    c) cuticle size
    d) the color of tinted hair

25. The section of hair that determines the length of the cut is the:
    a) parting
    b) guideline
    c) section
    d) graduation line

26. When hair falls naturally and each subsection is slightly shorter than the guide, it is called:
    a) blunt cutting
    b) undercutting
    c) layering
    d) notching

27. Scissors-over-comb is used to:
    a) create volume
    b) correct cowlicks
    c) create very short tapers
    d) leave length at the nape

28. Thinning hair with the shears is known as slithering or:
    a) shearing
    b) feathering
    c) blending
    d) effilating

29. An example of a fast rhythm pattern is:
    a) large curls
    b) one-length styles
    c) long waves
    d) tight curls

30. A narrow forehead may look wider using highlights at the:
    a) nape
    b) temples
    c) parting
    d) crown

31. The square facial type can be identified by the square jawline and:
    a) irregular hairline
    b) hollow cheeks
    c) narrow forehead
    d) straight hairline

32. Pinching or pushing ridges with fingers will create:
    a) underdirection of ridges
    b) splits
    c) overdirection of ridges
    d) uneven width of waves

33. The stationary part of a pin curl is the:
    a) curl
    b) stem
    c) wave
    d) base

34. With a side part hairstyle, the finger wave should begin on:
    a) the left side
    b) the heavy side
    c) the right side
    d) the light side

35. Always begin pin curls at the _____ end of a shaping.
    a) open
    b) bottom
    c) top
    d) circular

    D

36. Volume is determined by the size of the roller and:
    a) the number of rollers used
    b) the direction of the curl
    c) how it sits on its base
    d) the direction of the anchoring clips

    C

37. For the least amount of volume in a roller set, use the:
    a) on-base method
    b) one-half base method
    c) off-base method
    d) open-end method

    C

38. Cornrowing is done in the same fashion as:
    a) visible French braids
    b) overlapped braids
    c) invisible French braids
    d) regular braids

    A

39. The required temperature of heated thermal irons depends on:
    a) the type of irons used
    b) the hair texture
    c) the cosmetologist's speed
    d) the size of the heater

    B

40. For successful blow-dry styling, the air should be directed from the scalp area to the:
    a) floor
    b) root
    c) face
    d) hair ends

    D

41. A method of wrapping long hair for a permanent wave is the:
    a) double halo method
    b) dropped crown method
    c) piggyback method
    d) single halo method

    C

42. The main active ingredient in acid-balanced waving lotion is:
    a) ammonium thioglycolate
    b) sodium hydroxide
    c) glyceryl monothioglycolate
    d) hydrogen peroxide

    C

43. Cold waving lotion:
    a) hardens hair
    b) dries hair
    c) sets hair
    d) softens hair

    D

44. A benefit derived from alkaline perm lotion is:
    a) a softer curl
    b) slower processing time
    c) a strong curl pattern
    d) its gentleness for delicate hair

    A

45. The ability of the hair to absorb moisture is known as:
    a) porosity
    b) texture
    c) elasticity
    d) density

    A

46. When checking for an S-pattern, the hair must be unwound:
    a) 2 1/2 turns
    b) 2 turns
    c) 1 turn
    d) 1 1/2 turns

    D

47. The difference between a body wave and a perm is:
    a) if the hair is tinted
    b) the size of the rod used
    c) the solution used
    d) the amount of neutralizer used

    B

48. Fine-textured hair:
    a) is resistant to lightening
    b) has an average response to color
    c) may process darker when depositing color
    d) may process lighter when depositing color

    C

49. The warmth or coolness of a color is known as:
    a) level
    b) intensity
    c) depth
    d) tone

    B

50. Red, yellow, and blue are considered:
    a) warm colors
    b) secondary colors
    c) primary colors
    d) cool colors

    C

51. If a client has unwanted orange tones, use a haircolor with a:
    a) violet base
    b) blue base
    c) green base
    d) yellow base

    B

52. Temporary haircolor:
    a) makes a physical change
    b) requires a strand test
    c) penetrates the cortex
    d) lasts 4–6 shampoos

    C

53. Henna is a form of:
    a) semi-permanent color
    b) metallic dye
    c) oxidation tint
    d) vegetable tint

    D

54. Oxidation tints work by: 3\5
    a) coating the cuticle
    b) swelling the hair shaft
    c) coating the cortex
    d) becoming trapped in the cuticle

    B

55. When formulating for semi-permanent haircolor, half of the formula is:
    a) the client's skin tone
    b) the natural hair color
    c) the client's eye color
    d) the last color used

    B

56. The highest volume of peroxide used with lighteners is:
    a) 10
    b) 30
    c) 20   C
    d) 40

    D

57. Powder bleaches cannot be applied to:
    a) the scalp
    b) gray hair
    c) hair darker than a level 5
    d) hair darker than a level 3

    A

58. Lightener subsections should be:
    a) 1/2"
    b) 1/8"
    c) 1/4"
    d) 1"

    B

59. Fillers are used to equalize porosity and:
    a) open the cuticle
    b) diffuse melanin
    c) deposit a base color
    d) remove color buildup

    C

60. When using a sodium hydroxide relaxer, the client's scalp is protected with:
    a) gel
    b) stabilizer
    c) petroleum cream
    d) conditioner

    C

61. A hair relaxing treatment should be avoided when the client has a presence of:
    a) pityriasis
    b) scalp abrasions
    c) prior styling products
    d) excessive oils

    B

62. When performing a chemical blow-out, the hair must not be:
    a) colored
    b) lifted
    c) underrelaxed
    d) overrelaxed

    D

63. A soft-curl permanent should not be given to hair that is:
    a) relaxed with sodium hydroxide
    b) not ethnic hair
    c) relaxed with ammonium thioglycolate
    d) overly curly

    A

64. The temperature of a pressing comb should be adjusted to the hair's:
    a) cleanliness
    b) style
    c) texture
    d) length

    C

65. If the pressing comb is not hot enough, the hair will:
    a) require more pressure
    b) not straighten
    c) require more pressing oil
    d) need a double press

    B

66. The use of excess heat on gray, tinted, or lightened hair may:
    a) alter future hair growth
    b) make the hair wiry
    c) discolor the hair
    d) ruin the pressing comb

    C

67. The actual pressing or straightening of the hair is accomplished with the comb's:
    a) teeth
    b) back rod
    c) handle
    d) tail

    B

68. Human hair wigs can be distinguished from synthetic hair wigs by a:
    a) match test
    b) pull test
    c) predisposition test
    d) strand test

    A

69. Nail shapes should conform to the client's:
    a) fingertips
    b) nail bed
    c) hand size
    d) free edge

    A

70. To mend torn, broken, or split nails, and to fortify weak or fragile nails, the following service is recommended:
    a) an oil manicure
    b) cuticle pushing
    c) nail wrapping
    d) a basic manicure

    C

71. Pumice powder is likely to be an ingredient found in:
    a) cuticle cream
    c) hand cream
    b) dry nail polish
    d) nail abrasive

    _D_

72. A physician who specializes in foot care is a/an:
    a) pediatrician
    c) orthopedic surgeon
    b) podiatrist
    d) ophthalmologist

    _B_

73. The nail plate is also known as the:
    a) mantle
    c) free edge
    b) nail body
    d) nail bed

    _D_

74. The cuticle overlapping the lunula is the:
    a) hyponychium
    c) perionychium
    b) eponychium
    d) nail wall

    _B_

75. The deep fold of skin in which the nail root is embedded is the:
    a) lunula
    c) mantle
    b) nail wall
    d) nail groove

    C   _B_

76. An infectious and inflammatory condition of the tissues surrounding the nail is known as:
    a) onychatrophia
    c) onychia
    b) paronychia
    d) onychoptosis

    _B_

77. The only service you may perform on a client with nail fungus or nail mold is to:
    a) apply polish
    c) buff to a shine
    b) remove artificial nails
    d) refill the new growth

    _B_

78. The fixed attachment of one end of a muscle to a bone or tissue is known as the _____ of a muscle.
    a) joint
    c) point
    b) origin
    d) insertion

    _B_

79. Milia is a common skin disorder that occurs in skin texture that is:
    a) coarse
    c) fine
    b) oily
    d) soft

    L   _B_

80. Translucent powder is:
   a) darker than foundation
   b) colorless
   c) lighter than foundation
   d) the same color as foundation

   C

81. Eye tabbing involves:
   a) applying strip eyelashes
   b) applying individual lashes
   c) tinting eyelashes
   d) removing artificial lashes

   B

82. The skin is thickest on the:
   a) palms and soles
   b) abdomen
   c) buttocks
   d) thighs

   A

83. The growth of the epidermis starts in the stratum:
   a) lucidum
   b) germinativum
   c) corneum
   d) granulosum

   B

84. Sensory nerve fibers in the skin react to:
   a) light
   b) sound
   c) cold
   d) fear

   C

85. The study of the structure, functions, and disorders of the skin is known as:
   a) trichology
   b) etiology
   c) pathology
   d) dermatology

   D

86. After a wound heals, a _____ may develop.
   a) vesicle
   b) cicatrix
   c) carbuncle
   d) furuncle

   B

87. Anhidrosis means:
   a) lack of perspiration
   b) excessive perspiration
   c) foul-smelling perspiration
   d) normal perspiration

   A

88. Abnormal white patches on the skin are called:
   a) chloasma
   b) albinism
   c) leucoderma
   d) rosacea

   C

89. Cold wax is normally removed from the treatment area with:
   a) tweezers
   b) solvent
   c) cotton cloth
   d) gloves

   C

90. Tissue is a group of similar:
    a) hormones
    b) muscles
    c) connections
    d) cells

    D

91. Bones consist of about two-thirds mineral matter and one-third:
    a) animal matter
    b) liquid matter
    c) gaseous matter
    d) chemical matter

    570

    A

92. An ampere is a unit of electrical:
    a) usage
    b) resistance
    c) tension
    d) strength

    D

93. Treatment by means of light rays is called:
    a) heat treatment
    b) infrared treatment
    c) electrotherapy
    d) ultraviolet treatment

    C

    D

94. When two or more elements combine chemically in definite weight proportions, they form a new substance called a:
    a) mixture
    b) compound
    c) suspension
    d) solution

    B

95. The hydrophilic end of a shampoo molecule is attracted to:
    a) oil
    b) hair
    c) water
    d) conditioner

    C

96. Building maintenance and renovations are covered by:
    a) federal laws
    b) local ordinances
    c) state laws
    d) the department of licensing

    B

97. The largest expense item in a salon is:
    a) rent
    b) supplies
    c) salaries
    d) advertising

    C

98. Products that are sold to clients are:
    a) stock supplies
    b) retail supplies
    c) consumption supplies
    d) wholesale supplies

    B

99. A salon that is owned by stockholders and has a state charter is a/an:
    a) corporation
    b) private business
    c) partnership
    d) individual ownership

    A

100. When selecting the location for a salon, you should consider:

a) your personnel policies
b) the services you will offer
c) the number of staff to hire
d) direct competition

D

ANSWER KEY

YOUR PROFESSIONAL IMAGE ✓

1. B	10. B	19. A	28. D	37. B
2. C	11. A	20. D	29. C	38. D
3. C	12. B	21. C	30. D	39. D
4. B	13. A	22. D	31. B	40. C
5. D	14. D	23. A	32. B	41. C
6. B	15. C	24. B	33. A	42. B
7. D	16. B	25. C	34. C	43. A
8. D	17. C	26. C	35. B	
9. A	18. B	27. D	36. C	

BACTERIOLOGY ✓

1. C	7. C	13. B	19. B	25. B
2. B	8. B	14. C	20. C	26. A
3. A	9. A	15. A	21. B	27. D
4. D	10. C	16. B	22. C	
5. B	11. B	17. C	23. D	
6. C	12. A	18. B	24. A	

DECONTAMINATION AND INFECTION CONTROL

1. B	8. D	15. B	22. B	29. B
2. D	9. B	16. C	23. A	30. C
3. C	10. B	17. B	24. D	31. D
4. D	11. C	18. A	25. B	32. A
5. B	12. D	19. C	26. A	33. B
6. B	13. C	20. D	27. B	34. C
7. B	14. B	21. D	28. D	35. C

PROPERTIES OF THE HAIR AND SCALP

1. C	23. D	45. B	67. B	89. D
2. D	24. A	46. D	68. A	90. C
3. B	25. D	47. B	69. A	91. D
4. B	26. C	48. B	70. C	92. A
5. A	27. D	49. C	71. B	93. B
6. B	28. D	50. D	72. C	94. B
7. C	29. A	51. B	73. A	95. D
8. A	30. C	52. A	74. D	96. B
9. B	31. C	53. C	75. C	97. C
10. B	32. D	54. B	76. D	98. D
11. D	33. A	55. B	77. C	99. B
12. A	34. B	56. D	78. B	100. B
13. B	35. D	57. D	79. C	101. D
14. C	36. B	58. B	80. B	102. B
15. B	37. D	59. C	81. D	103. D
16. B	38. C	60. D	82. C	104. B
17. D	39. D	61. B	83. C	105. C
18. A	40. B	62. D	84. A	106. D
19. B	41. D	63. C	85. C	107. C
20. C	42. D	64. C	86. B	108. D
21. C	43. D	65. B	87. A	109. B
22. B	44. C	66. D	88. B	110. D

DRAPING

1. B	3. C	5. C	7. B	9. D
2. B	4. A	6. B	8. A	10. D

SHAMPOOING, RINSING, AND CONDITIONING

1. B	6. B	11. D	16. A	21. D
2. C	7. D	12. C	17. A	22. B
3. B	8. A	13. B	18. A	23. A
4. A	9. A	14. B	19. B	24. D
5. D	10. B	15. C	20. D	25. C

HAIRCUTTING

1. B	9. D	17. B	25. B	33. D
2. C	10. C	18. C	26. C	34. B
3. C	11. B	19. B	27. A	35. B
4. D	12. C	20. D	28. C	36. C
5. A	13. A	21. B	29. C	37. D
6. C	14. C	22. B	30. B	38. A
7. B	15. D	23. C	31. B	39. D
8. B	16. A	24. A	32. A	40. B

ARTISTRY IN HAIRSTYLING

1. B	8. B	15. B	22. A	29. C
2. D	9. C	16. C	23. D	30. A
3. C	10. A	17. D	24. C	31. D
4. D	11. D	18. B	25. D	32. B
5. A	12. B	19. B	26. C	33. C
6. C	13. D	20. A	27. B	34. A
7. B	14. A	21. D	28. D	35. D

WET HAIRSTYLING

1. B	10. A	19. D	28. D	37. C
2. A	11. A	20. B	29. C	38. B
3. C	12. C	21. B	30. B	39. B
4. B	13. D	22. C	31. C	40. C
5. C	14. B	23. D	32. D	41. C
6. D	15. A	24. A	33. B	42. A
7. D	16. B	25. B	34. B	
8. B	17. B	26. D	35. A	
9. B	18. C	27. B	36. B	

THERMAL HAIRSTYLING

1. B	7. C	13. A	19. D	25. C
2. A	8. B	14. C	20. C	26. C
3. C	9. C	15. C	21. B	27. D
4. A	10. B	16. C	22. A	28. D
5. B	11. D	17. B	23. D	29. D
6. D	12. B	18. C	24. B	30. B

PERMANENT WAVING

1. D	12. D	23. A	34. C	45. B
2. A	13. C	24. B	35. C	46. B
3. C	14. B	25. B	36. A	47. D
4. B	15. D	26. C	37. B	48. C
5. B	16. A	27. C	38. D	49. A
6. A	17. B	28. D	39. D	50. B
7. D	18. C	29. D	40. A	51. B
8. D	19. A	30. B	41. B	52. C
9. A	20. A	31. B	42. A	
10. B	21. C	32. C	43. A	
11. C	22. D	33. D	44. C	

HAIRCOLORING ✓

1. C	21. C	41. C	61. D	81. B
2. B	22. B	42. D	62. A	82. D
3. A	23. D	43. D	63. C	83. B
4. D	24. B	44. B	64. D	84. A
5. C	25. B	45. A	65. B	85. D
6. B	26. A	46. B	66. C	86. A
7. A	27. C	47. D	67. B	87. B
8. D	28. D	48. C	68. D	88. B
9. C	29. A	49. B	69. C	89. A
10. D	30. B	50. D	70. A	90. A
11. C	31. B	51. C	71. B	91. B
12. A	32. D	52. A	72. C	92. C
13. D	33. C	53. B	73. A	93. B
14. B	34. A	54. A	74. B	94. C
15. D	35. B	55. C	75. C	95. A
16. A	36. C	56. B	76. D	96. B
17. C	37. B	57. D	77. B	97. C
18. B	38. D	58. B	78. D	98. D
19. D	39. A	59. A	79. A	99. D
20. C	40. D	60. B	80. C	100. C

CHEMICAL HAIR RELAXING AND SOFT-CURL PERMANENT

1. C	8. D	15. A	22. D	29. A
2. A	9. B	16. D	23. B	30. C
3. D	10. D	17. B	24. C	31. A
4. C	11. C	18. B	25. A	32. A
5. D	12. B	19. D	26. B	33. C
6. B	13. C	20. B	27. D	34. A
7. D	14. B	21. C	28. B	35. B

THERMAL HAIR STRAIGHTENING

1. B	8. B	15. B	22. A	29. C
2. B	9. A	16. D	23. B	30. D
3. C	10. C	17. B	24. C	31. B
4. B	11. B	18. C	25. B	32. A
5. D	12. D	19. A	26. D	33. C
6. A	13. B	20. C	27. A	34. B
7. A	14. C	21. B	28. D	

THE ARTISTRY OF ARTIFICIAL HAIR

1. C	4. A	7. B	10. B	13. C
2. D	5. A	8. C	11. A	14. B
3. B	6. C	9. D	12. D	15. D

MANICURING AND PEDICURING

1. C	10. A	19. A	28. C	37. B
2. B	11. C	20. C	29. A	38. B
3. C	12. B	21. C	30. C	39. C
4. A	13. D	22. D	31. C	40. D
5. B	14. A	23. A	32. B	41. B
6. B	15. C	24. D	33. B	42. C
7. A	16. B	25. C	34. D	43. B
8. B	17. C	26. D	35. A	44. D
9. A	18. D	27. D	36. C	45. B

THE NAIL AND ITS DISORDERS

1. A	11. D	21. A	31. B	41. C
2. B	12. B	22. B	32. B	42. C
3. D	13. B	23. D	33. A	43. B
4. C	14. C	24. A	34. C	44. B
5. A	15. B	25. C	35. B	45. B
6. C	16. B	26. B	36. C	46. A
7. D	17. D	27. C	37. A	47. D
8. D	18. C	28. C	38. C	48. C
9. B	19. B	29. A	39. B	49. D
10. A	20. D	30. D	40. B	50. B

THEORY OF MASSAGE

1. D	5. C	9. A	13. A	17. D
2. D	6. D	10. D	14. B	18. B
3. A	7. C	11. C	15. D	19. D
4. C	8. B	12. B	16. B	20. A

FACIALS

1. C	6. C	11. D	16. B	21. C
2. C	7. D	12. C	17. D	22. D
3. A	8. B	13. B	18. C	23. D
4. C	9. B	14. A	19. C	24. C
5. D	10. C	15. B	20. B	25. D

FACIAL MAKEUP

1. D	6. B	11. C	16. B	21. D
2. B	7. A	12. D	17. C	22. A
3. B	8. B	13. C	18. B	23. A
4. A	9. A	14. B	19. A	24. C
5. D	10. B	15. B	20. B	

THE SKIN AND ITS DISORDERS

1. C	19. B	37. D	55. A	73. C
2. C	20. B	38. D	56. B	74. B
3. B	21. D	39. C	57. C	75. B
4. B	22. D	40. C	58. A	76. B
5. A	23. B	41. D	59. A	77. B
6. B	24. C	42. C	60. D	78. A
7. C	25. C	43. D	61. C	79. D
8. D	26. C	44. B	62. C	80. D
9. B	27. A	45. B	63. C	81. C
10. B	28. C	46. D	64. A	82. B
11. B	29. B	47. C	65. C	83. C
12. B	30. B	48. C	66. C	84. B
13. C	31. B	49. B	67. C	85. C
14. A	32. A	50. C	68. B	86. C
15. B	33. B	51. A	69. D	87. A
16. C	34. B	52. B	70. B	88. D
17. B	35. C	53. D	71. C	89. B
18. A	36. C	54. C	72. A	90. C

REMOVING UNWANTED HAIR

1. D	5. C	9. B	13. C	17. D
2. C	6. B	10. D	14. A	18. B
3. A	7. C	11. D	15. C	19. C
4. B	8. B	12. C	16. D	20. A

CELLS, ANATOMY, AND PHYSIOLOGY

1. B	21. C	41. A	61. D	81. C
2. A	22. C	42. D	62. A	82. C
3. C	23. D	43. A	63. B	83. B
4. D	24. A	44. B	64. A	84. C
5. A	25. B	45. C	65. C	85. A
6. D	26. B	46. B	66. A	86. A
7. A	27. C	47. A	67. A	87. B
8. D	28. D	48. B	68. C	88. A
9. D	29. C	49. C	69. B	89. B
10. C	30. C	50. D	70. D	90. D
11. B	31. B	51. B	71. C	91. A
12. C	32. B	52. D	72. D	92. C
13. C	33. A	53. C	73. B	93. A
14. B	34. A	54. D	74. A	94. B
15. C	35. B	55. C	75. C	95. A
16. A	36. C	56. D	76. A	96. B
17. B	37. A	57. A	77. A	97. C
18. B	38. B	58. B	78. C	98. D
19. A	39. B	59. B	79. B	99. C
20. B	40. C	60. B	80. D	100. B

ELECTRICITY AND LIGHT THERAPY √

1. D	7. D	13. D	19. C	25. D
2. A	8. C	14. C	20. B	26. D
3. A	9. A	15. A	21. B	27. B
4. B	10. B	16. C	22. D	28. D
5. B	11. D	17. D	23. B	29. B
6. B	12. C	18. A	24. D	30. D

CHEMISTRY

1. A	10. C	19. B	28. C	37. D
2. B	11. C	20. D	29. B	38. B
3. D	12. B	21. C	30. C	39. A
4. A	13. A	22. B	31. A	40. D
5. A	14. D	23. A	32. A	41. C
6. A	15. A	24. C	33. B	42. A
7. C	16. A	25. B	34. B	43. B
8. B	17. C	26. D	35. A	44. A
9. D	18. B	27. C	36. C	45. C

THE SALON BUSINESS

1. D	9. B	17. D	25. C	33. A
2. A	10. B	18. B	26. A	34. C
3. B	11. D	19. A	27. D	35. B
4. B	12. A	20. C	28. C	36. A
5. A	13. C	21. C	29. D	37. D
6. C	14. B	22. B	30. D	38. B
7. B	15. D	23. C	31. B	39. D
8. A	16. C	24. A	32. A	40. A

TEST 1

1. A	21. A	41. A	61. B	81. B
2. C	22. D	42. D	62. A	82. A
3. B	23. B	43. B	63. D	83. B
4. B	24. B	44. A	64. B	84. C
5. C	25. C	45. B	65. C	85. D
6. D	26. C	46. D	66. B	86. D
7. B	27. D	47. B	67. A	87. C
8. B	28. B	48. A	68. D	88. B
9. C	29. D	49. D	69. D	89. A
10. B	30. B	50. C	70. C	90. B
11. B	31. C	51. D	71. D	91. B
12. A	32. D	52. C	72. A	92. D
13. B	33. B	53. A	73. C	93. A
14. A	34. C	54. D	74. A	94. A
15. C	35. A	55. C	75. C	95. B
16. B	36. B	56. B	76. B	96. C
17. B	37. C	57. A	77. C	97. C
18. D	38. D	58. B	78. D	98. D
19. A	39. B	59. D	79. B	99. A
20. B	40. C	60. B	80. C	100. B

TEST 2

1. C	21. D	41. C	61. B	81. B
2. A	22. B	42. C	62. D	82. A
3. B	23. A	43. D	63. A	83. B
4. D	24. D	44. C	64. C	84. C
5. A	25. B	45. A	65. B	85. D
6. C	26. C	46. A	66. C	86. B
7. B	27. C	47. B	67. B	87. A
8. B	28. D	48. C	68. A	88. C
9. D	29. D	49. D	69. A	89. C
10. C	30. B	50. C	70. C	90. D
11. C	31. D	51. B	71. D	91. A
12. B	32. C	52. A	72. B	92. D
13. B	33. D	53. D	73. D	93. C
14. D	34. B	54. B	74. B	94. B
15. D	35. A	55. B	75. C	95. C
16. B	36. C	56. C	76. B	96. B
17. D	37. C	57. A	77. B	97. C
18. A	38. A	58. B	78. B	98. B
19. C	39. B	59. C	79. C	99. A
20. B	40. D	60. C	80. B	100. D

dry crystals – ch 12
324

Natural hair color categories – ch 12
274 – 277

pg 54-55 Hair Cycles

pg 59 |
277
455

Ch 22 Methods of Hair removal
Ch 23
Endo / Exo (227)
└ heat